Osteoarthritis

Guest Editor

DAVID J. HUNTER, MBBS, PhD

CLINICS IN GERIATRIC MEDICINE

www.geriatric.theclinics.com

August 2010 • Volume 26 • Number 3

SAUNDERS an imprint of ELSEVIER, Inc.

MT

W.B. SAUNDERS COMPANY
A Division of Elsevier Inc.

1600 John F. Kennedy Blvd., Suite 1800. Philadelphia, Pennsylvania 19103-2899

http://www.theclinics.com

CLINICS IN GERIATRIC MEDICINE Volume 26, Number 3
August 2010 ISSN 0749–0690, ISBN-13: 978-1-4377-2453-0

Editor: Yonah Korngold
Developmental Editor: Donald Mumford

Clinics in Geriatric Medicine (ISSN 0749-0690) is published quarterly by Elsevier Inc., 360 Park Avenue South, New York, NY 10010-1710. Months of issue are February, May, August, and November. Business and Editorial Offices: 1600 John F. Kennedy Blvd., Suite 1800, Philadelphia, PA 191023-2899. Periodicals postage paid at New York, NY, and additional mailing offices. Subscription prices is $225.00 per year (US individuals), $388.00 per year (US institutions), $293.00 per year (Canadian individuals), $484.00 per year (Canadian institutions), $311.00 per year (foreign individuals) and $484.00 per year (foreign institutions). Foreign air speed delivery is included in all *Clinics* subscription prices. All prices are subject to change without notice. POSTMASTER: Send address changes to *Clinics in Geriatric Medicine,* Elsevier Health Sciences Division, Subscription Customer Service, 3251 Riverport Lane, Maryland Heights, MO 63043. Telephone: 1-800-654-2452 (U.S. and Canada); 314-447-8871 (outside U.S. and Canada). Fax: 314-447-8029. E-mail: journalscustomerservice-usa@elsevier.com (for print support) or journalsonlinesupport-usa@elsevier.com (for online support).

Reprints. For copies of 100 or more, of articles in this publication, please contact the Commercial Reprints Department, Elsevier Inc., 360 Park Avenue South, New York, New York 10010-1710. Tel.: (212) 633-3812; Fax: (212) 462-1935, email: reprints@elsevier.com.

Clinics in Geriatric Medicine is covered in *MEDLINE/PubMed (Index Medicus), EMBASE/Excerpta Medica, Current Contents/Clinical Medicine (CC/CM),* and the *Cumulative Index to Nursing & Allied Health Literature.*

Printed in the United States of America.

8/22/11

Contributors

GUEST EDITOR

DAVID J. HUNTER, MBBS, PhD, FRACP
Department of Rheumatology, Northern Clinical School, University of Sydney, Sydney, Australia; Division of Research, New England Baptist Hospital, Boston, Massachusetts

AUTHORS

JAMES V. BONO, MD
Clinical Professor in Orthopaedic Surgery, Tufts University School of Medicine, New England Baptist Hospital, Boston, Massachusetts

PAUL DIEPPE, BSc, MD, FRCP, FFPH
Chair of Clinical Education Research, Peninsula Medical School, Universities of Exeter and Plymouth, United Kingdom

MICHAEL DOHERTY, MA, MD, FRCP
Professor of Rheumatology, University of Nottingham; Academic Rheumatology, Nottingham, United Kingdom

K. DOUGLAS GROSS, PT, ScD
Assistant Professor, Graduate Programs in Physical Therapy, MGH Institute of Health Professions, Charlestown Navy Yard, Boston, Massachusetts

WILLIAM H. GRUBER, PhD
Former Chief Information Officer of the Risk Management Foundation, Harvard Medical Institutions; Co-inventor of the Chief Information Officer concept; Former academic appointments at the MIT Sloan School of Management, Harvard Business School, Boston College; Northeastern University, Boston, Massachusetts

WILLIAM F. HARVEY, MD, MSc
Assistant Professor of Medicine, Division of Rheumatology, Tufts Medical Center; Division of Research, New England Baptist Hospital, Boston, Massachusetts

DAVID J. HUNTER, MBBS, PhD, FRACP
Department of Rheumatology, Northern Clinical School, University of Sydney, Sydney, Australia; Division of Research, New England Baptist Hospital, Boston, Massachusetts

ALAN M. JETTE, PhD, PT
Department of Health Policy and Management, Health and Disability Research Institute, Boston University School of Public Health, Boston, Massachusetts

JOANNE M. JORDAN, MD, MPH
Thurston Arthritis Research Center, University of North Carolina, Chapel Hill, North Carolina

NANCY LATHAM, PhD, PT
Research Assistant Professor, Health and Disability Research Institute, Boston University School of Public Health, Boston, Massachusetts

CHIUNG-JU LIU, PhD, OTR
Assistant Professor, Department of Occupational Therapy, School of Health and Rehabilitation Sciences, Indiana University, Indianapolis, Indiana

RICHARD F. LOESER, MD
Professor of Internal Medicine, Section of Molecular Medicine; Director of Translational Research, Wake Forest University School of Medicine, Winston-Salem, North Carolina

CHRISTINE M. MCDONOUGH, PhD, PT
Department of Health Policy and Management, Health and Disability Research Institute, Boston University School of Public Health, Boston, Massachusetts; The Dartmouth Institute for Health Policy and Clinical Practice, Dartmouth College, Hanover, New Hampshire

STEPHEN P. MESSIER, PhD
Professor, Department of Health and Exercise Science, Wake Forest University, Winston-Salem, North Carolina

CLAIRE E. ROBBINS, PT
New England Baptist Hospital, Tufts University, Boston, Massachusetts

CARL T. TALMO, MD
Assistant Clinical Professor in Orthopaedic Surgery, Tufts University School of Medicine, New England Baptist Hospital, Boston, Massachusetts

YUQING ZHANG, DSc
Clinical Epidemiology Research and Training Unit, Boston University School of Medicine, Boston, Massachusetts

Contents

Osteoarthritis (OA) is the most common joint disorder in the United States. Symptomatic knee OA occurs in 10% men and 13% in women aged 60 years or older. The number of people affected with symptomatic OA is likely to increase due to the aging of the population and the obesity epidemic. OA has a multifactorial etiology, and can be considered the product of an interplay between systemic and local factors. Old age, female gender, overweight and obesity, knee injury, repetitive use of joints, bone density, muscle weakness, and joint laxity all play roles in the development of joint OA, particularly in the weight-bearing joints. Modifying these factors may reduce the risk of OA and prevent subsequent pain and disability.

Osteoarthritis (OA) is the most common cause of chronic disability in older adults. Although classically considered a "wear and tear" degenerative condition of articular joints, recent studies have demonstrated an inflammatory component to OA that includes increased activity of several cytokines and chemokines in joint tissues that drive production of matrix-degrading enzymes. Rather than directly causing OA, aging changes in the musculoskeletal system contribute to the development of OA by making the joint more susceptible to the effects of other OA risk factors that include abnormal biomechanics, joint injury, genetics, and obesity. Age-related sarcopenia and increased bone turnover may also contribute to the development of OA. Understanding the basic mechanisms by which aging affects joint tissues should provide new targets for slowing or preventing the development of OA.

This article uses the Disablement Model conceptual framework to guide an analysis of the importance of osteoarthritis (OA) in the development of disability. The Disablement Model describes the development and progression of disablement from impairments to specific functional limitations and disability, and the hypothesized role of predisposing risk factors, extra-individual factors, and intra-individual factors. A wide range of population and clinical studies have characterized the unequivocal contribution of arthritis to the development of functional limitations and disability. Evidence overwhelmingly supports a significant, moderate independent contribution of arthritis to the onset and progression of functional limitations and disability. With respect to important risk factors for the development of functional limitations and disability among those with OA, the evidence provides strong support for the role of physical impairments along with other predisposing and intra-individual factors such as age, body mass index, obesity, lack of exercise, comorbid conditions, depression, and depressive symptoms. Extra-individual factors included need for aids and assistance, and lack of access to public or private transportation. Future disablement research must clarify the causal mechanisms behind a potential risk factor's impact on disability and delineate the interplay between and among the various hypothesized steps in the disablement process.

Evidence-based guidelines have the potential to improve the quality of health care by promoting interventions of proven benefit and discouraging unnecessary, ineffective, or harmful interventions. Recent years have seen the development of several evidence-based guidelines developed for osteoarthritis (OA) management. There is some consistency in the numerous guidelines that are available for OA management, yet despite some dissemination attempts, clinical practice does not reflect these recommendations. Current clinical practice reflects a multitude of factors, including clinician and patient preference and health care system support. Similarly, guidelines are frequently prescribed independent of context and thus implementation can be challenging. Future efforts to guide management of OA of the hip or knee are better directed towards implementing practices known to be effective in a context-dependent manner to optimize health care quality.

Osteoarthritis (OA) is not an easy condition to manage. It is very heterogeneous, has an unpredictable natural history, and has variable effects on health status. A wide range of management options is available to OA patients and their health care advisors. Guidelines help the clinician through this complexity. There are many similarities in the advice offered by different guidelines, suggesting a good deal of consensus on what should and should not be offered to patients with OA. Several authoritative international guidelines on OA management have appeared in recent years. In this article the authors evaluate the United Kingdom National Institute for Clinical Excellence guidelines as a contemporary tool to assess the context within which care is delivered and as the basis for discussion on the gap between evidence and practice.

This article describes the dysfunctional delivery of existing conservative care practices in the treatment of osteoarthritis (OA) within the context of a dynamic environment of health reform. It is written from the patient perspective of one of the authors who is afflicted with OA and with the added clinical view of a rheumatologist. The authors envision benefits of more cost-effective care, a decrease in the impact of chronic illness on the financial viability of the United States, and an improvement in the quality of care provided to patients. These benefits can be achieved with tested innovations organized within the integrated delivery system described in this article.

THE CLINICS ARE NOW AVAILABLE ONLINE!

Access your subscription at:
www.theclinics.com

Preface

Osteoarthritis

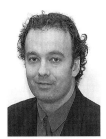

David J. Hunter, MBBS, PhD, FRACP
Guest Editor

Osteoarthritis (OA) is the leading cause of disability among older adults. It is already an incredibly prevalent condition and one that is becoming even more prevalent with the combined effects of an aging and increasingly obese society. In this context, this issue of *Clinics in Geriatric Medicine* is timely, as we envision this increasingly prevalent disabling condition in an era when health care expenditure is increasingly scrutinized.

With these societal trends, new insights are developing into the pervasive disease we know as OA. Consideration of the impact of this condition in our society requires an understanding of the incidence and prevalence of this disease. Drs Zhang and Jordan provide a thoughtful appraisal of the epidemiology of OA, illuminating us on how we define OA (both radiographically and symptomatically), the prevalence and incidence of OA, and risk factors for OA.

Dr Loeser provides a thoughtful review of the biology of OA and the relationship between aging and the development of OA. We now conceptualize OA as a disease of the whole joint organ. Critically, the disease is no longer viewed as a passive, degenerative disorder but rather an active disease process driven primarily by mechanical factors. In addition, an inflammatory component to OA that includes increased activity of a number of cytokines and chemokines in joint tissues drives production of matrix-degrading enzymes. Rather than directly causing OA, aging changes in the musculoskeletal system contribute to the development of OA by making the joint more susceptible to the effects of other OA risk factors that include abnormal biomechanics, joint injury, genetics, and obesity.

As the leading cause of disability in older adults, it is critical that we consider the genesis of this disability. Within the disablement model conceptual framework, Drs McDonough and Jette review the significant contribution of OA to the onset and progression of functional limitations and disability. With respect to important risk factors for the development of functional limitations and disability among those with OA, there is strong support for the role of physical impairments along with other

Dr Hunter is funded by an Australian Research Council Future Fellowship.

Clin Geriatr Med 26 (2010) xi–xiii
doi:10.1016/j.cger.2010.06.001 **geriatric.theclinics.com**

predisposing and intraindividual factors, such as age, body mass index, obesity, lack of exercise, comorbid conditions, depression, and depressive symptoms.

Sir William Osler, considered the "Father of Modern Medicine," once said, "When an arthritis patient walks in the front door, I feel like leaving by the back door." For many clinicians this attitude still holds true; however, there is much the interested clinician can do rather than nihilistic waiting. I provide a narrative review that outlines the management of the patient with OA, how standard clinical practice diverges from what is recommended, and some key challenges facing clinicians with regard to optimizing quality-of-care delivery in OA.

No one denies that the management of OA is a challenge and the frequency with which expert groups develop recommendations both highlights this challenge and at times further complicates it. Unfortunately, despite what many guidelines would make you believe, there is not one size or prescription that fits all. OA management needs to be individualized and patient centered. Drs Doherty and Dieppe review the gap between evidence and practice and provide reasons for this separation. Their thoughtful review provides stimulation to clinicians to improve their care of older people with OA.

The challenge facing clinicians is dwarfed by the experience that persons with OA have to face. Any person with a chronic illness faces a personal daily battle with the condition itself that, in the case of OA, is further compounded by a nihilistic "broken" health care system. I have had the distinct pleasure of coauthoring a review with Dr William Gruber on the current state of OA management in our health care system and progressive steps that can be taken in this era of health care reform.

For the practicing clinician, arming themselves with evidence for disease management is critical and the ensuing articles, particularly those on strength training, obesity management, and device use, are critical, as these are far too frequently overlooked in clinical practice. It is important that symptomatic improvement serve the purpose of increasing tolerance for functional activity. Ultimately, an efficacious treatment for any progressive disorder should also control the factors and forces that drive disease progression. These sections highlight this need.

Drs Latham and Liu summarize the findings of randomized controlled trials of progressive resistance strength training by older people with OA. Their results suggest that strength training has particularly strong functional benefits for older adults with OA. They go on to discuss how older adults with OA will benefit from a strength training program and how clinicians should encourage and prescribe participation in exercise training programs.

The impact of, and mechanisms by which, obesity affects OA are of great concern at both societal and individual levels. Dr Messier, a master in this field, reviews the physiologic and mechanical consequences of obesity on older adults with OA: the effects of long-term exercise and weight-loss interventions, the most effective non-pharmacologic treatments for obesity; and the usefulness, practicality, and feasibility of prescribing these in clinical practice.

The goal of many noninvasive devices for OA is to alter joint biomechanics in such a way as to limit regional exposure to potentially damaging and provocative mechanical stresses. Because of their targeted intention, optimal prescription of most noninvasive devices requires that we first specify which mechanical stresses we wish to reduce. Dr Gross lends his expertise and reviews several of the most important devices currently used in the treatment of OA.

Ultimately many patients seek assistance for pain relief in the form of pharmacologic intervention. Dr Harvey and I review the current trends and controversies related to pharmacologic management, including the use of oral, topical, and injectable agents. Before recommending any pharmacologic intervention, it is important to reconcile the delicate balance between effectiveness and toxicity.

Failing prior interventions, OA surgery may become necessary. Although the indications for arthroscopy have narrowed, joint replacement continues to play a pivotal role in disease management. Drs Talmo, Robbins, and Bono review the role and indications for joint replacement in older adults. They highlight the perioperative issues, including monitoring, preventative measures, and complications, that are critical to consider in adequately managing joint replacement in older adults.

Looking forward we are reminded by the late Sir Henry Tizard that "The secret of science is to ask the right question, and it is the choice of problem more than anything else that marks the man of genius in the scientific world." We have been afforded an opportunity to study a much maligned disease that is rapidly evolving. Let us learn from the insights our research is providing to focus even more on important modifiable risk factors, such as mechanics and obesity, as we develop the therapeutic armamentarium of the twenty-first century. Assuming we maintain a meaningful motivation with the patient at the forefront of our minds, we have an opportunity to make a difference in millions of people's lives. I look forward to the evolution ahead.

I would sincerely like to thank my friends and colleagues for their valuable contributions to this issue. They were a pleasure to work with and I am sure you will see from the contents that their respective manuscripts reflect wonderful insight and appraisal of a complex and developing field.

David J. Hunter, MBBS, PhD, FRACP
Department of Rheumatology, Northern Clinical School
University of Sydney, 2065, Sydney, Australia
Division of Research, New England Baptist Hospital
125 Parker Hill Avenue, Boston, MA 02120, USA
Rheumatology Department, Level 4, Block 4
Royal North Shore Hospital, St Leonards 2065
New South Wales, Australia

E-mail address:
David.Hunter@sydney.edu.au

Epidemiology of Osteoarthritis

Yuqing Zhang, DSc[a],*, Joanne M. Jordan, MD, MPH[b]

KEYWORDS

• Osteoarthritis • Weight-bearing joints • Risk factors

Osteoarthritis (OA) is the most common joint disorder in the United States.[1] Among adults 60 years of age or older the prevalence of symptomatic knee OA is approximately 10% in men and 13% in women.[2] The number of people affected with symptomatic OA is likely to increase due to the aging of the population and the obesity epidemic.

Pain from OA is a key symptom in the decision to seek medical care and is an important antecedent to disability.[3] Because of its high prevalence and the frequent disability that accompanies disease in major joints such as the knee and hip, OA accounts for more difficulty with climbing stairs and walking than any other disease.[4] OA is also the most common reason for total hip and total knee replacement.[5] The rapid increase in the prevalence of this already common disease suggests that OA will have a growing impact on health care and public health systems in the future.[6]

DEFINING OSTEOARTHRITIS

Epidemiologic principles can be used to describe the distribution of OA in the population and to examine risk factors for its occurrence and progression. For the purpose of epidemiologic investigation, OA can be defined pathologically, radiographically, or clinically. Radiographic OA has long been considered the reference standard, and multiple ways to define radiographic disease have been devised. The most common method for radiographic definition is the Kellgren-Lawrence (K/L) radiographic grading scheme and atlas. which has been in use for over 4 decades. This overall joint scoring system grades OA in 5 levels from 0 to 4, defining OA by the presence of a definite osteophyte (Grade ≥ 2), and more severe grades by the presumed successive appearance of joint space narrowing, sclerosis, cysts, and deformity.[7] Other radiographic metrics including semiquantitative examination of individual radiographic features, such as osteophytes and joint space narrowing, or the direct measurement

[a] Clinical Epidemiology Research and Training Unit, Boston University School of Medicine, 650 Albany Street, Suite x200, Boston, MA 02118, USA
[b] Thurston Arthritis Research Center, University of North Carolina, 3300 Doc J. Thurston Jr Building, CB #7280, Chapel Hill, NC 27599-7289, USA
* Corresponding author.
E-mail address: yuqing@bu.edu

Clin Geriatr Med 26 (2010) 355–369
doi:10.1016/j.cger.2010.03.001
0749-0690/10/$ – see front matter © 2010 Elsevier Inc. All rights reserved.

of the interbone distance as an indicator of the joint space width in the knees and hips, are used to investigate progression in epidemiologic studies and clinical trials of disease-modifying therapies.[8,9] More sensitive imaging methods using magnetic resonance imaging (MRI) can visualize multiple structures in a joint and are undergoing evaluation for their role in defining OA and for their usefulness in detecting the effects of potential disease-modifying interventions more quickly than is possible with conventional radiographs.[10,11]

Studies of OA in people who have joint symptoms may be more clinically relevant, because not all persons who have radiographic OA have clinical disease, and not all persons who have joint symptoms demonstrate radiographic OA.[12] Each set of clinical and radiographic criteria may yield slightly different groups of subjects defined as having OA.[12]

PREVALENCE AND INCIDENCE OF OSTEOARTHRITIS

The prevalence of OA varies according to the definition of OA, the specific joint(s) under study, and the characteristics of the study population. The age-standardized prevalence of radiographic knee OA in adults age 45 years or older was 19.2% among the participants in the Framingham Study and 27.8% in the Johnston County Osteoarthritis Project.[6] In the third National Health and Nutrition Examination Survey (NHANES III), approximately 37% of participants older than 60 years had radiographic knee OA.[6]

Age-standardized prevalence of radiographic hand OA was 27.2% among the Framingham participants. Radiographic hip OA was less common than hand or knee OA. For example, about 7% of women age 65 years or older in the Study of Osteoporotic Fractures had radiographic hip OA. However, prevalence of hip OA was much higher in Johnston County, with 27% of subjects at least 45 years old demonstrating radiographic evidence of K/L grade 2 or higher OA.[6] Potential explanations for the differences between these studies relate to differences in study populations, definitions of OA, distribution of risk factors for disease, and radiographic readers.

Symptomatic OA is generally defined by the presence of pain, aching, or stiffness in a joint with radiographic OA. The age-standardized prevalence of symptomatic hand and knee OA is 6.8% and 4.9%, respectively, in Framingham subjects age 26 years or older. However, prevalence of symptomatic knee OA was 16.7% among subjects age 45 or older in the Johnston County Osteoarthritis Project, much higher than that reported in the Framingham Study. About 9% of subjects in the Johnston County study had symptomatic hip OA.[6] There is a paucity of meaningful data on the cumulative incidence of developing OA. Here, the length of time over which the risk of OA is calculated is critical but is not always clearly specified or known. Further, because OA is a chronic disease occurring mostly among the elderly, competing risk or death from other diseases makes direct estimation of the cumulative incidence of OA difficult.

Oliveria and colleagues[13] reported the age- and sex-standardized incidence rates of symptomatic hip, knee, and hand OA to be 88, 240, and 100 per 100,000 person-years, respectively, in participants in a Massachusetts health maintenance organization, and the incidence rates of symptomatic OA of either hand or knee, or hip increased rapidly around age 50 and then leveled off after age 70 (**Fig. 1**). Murphy and colleagues[14] estimated the lifetime risk of developing symptomatic knee OA to be about 40% in men and 47% in women. Such a risk rises to 60% in subjects with body mass index (BMI; calculated as the weight in kilograms divided by height in meters squared) of 30 or higher.

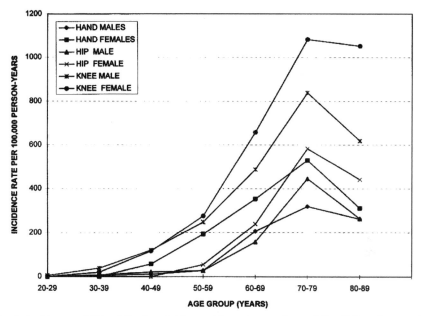

Fig. 1. Incidence of OA of the hand, hip, and knee in members of the Fallon Community Health Plan, 1991 to 1992, by age and sex. (*From* Oliveria SA, Felson DT, Reed JI, et al. Incidence of symptomatic hand, hip, and knee osteoarthritis among patients in a health maintenance organization. Arthritis Rheum 1995;38:1139; with permission.)

RISK FACTORS FOR OSTEOARTHRITIS

OA has a multifactorial etiology, and can be considered the product of an interplay between systemic and local factors as shown in **Fig. 2.**[1] For example, a person may have an inherited predisposition to develop OA but may only develop it if an insult to the joint has occurred. The relative importance of risk factors may vary for different joints, for different stages of the disease, for the development as opposed to the progression of disease, and for radiographic versus symptomatic disease. There is even some evidence suggesting that risk factors may act differently according to individual radiographic features, such as osteophytes and joint space narrowing.[1] Whether some of these differences are genuine or are spurious results of different study populations, definition of risk factors and OA, statistical power, or analytical methods is open to debate.

SYSTEMIC RISK FACTORS FOR OSTEOARTHRITIS
Age

Age is a one of the strongest risk factors for OA of all joints.[1,6,15] The increase in the prevalence and incidence of OA with age probably is a consequence of cumulative exposure to various risk factors and biologic changes that occur with aging that may make a joint less able to cope with adversity, such as cartilage thinning, weak muscle strength, poor proprioception, and oxidative damage.

Gender and Hormones

Women not only are more likely to have OA than men, they also have more severe OA.[16] The definite increase in OA in women around the time of menopause has led

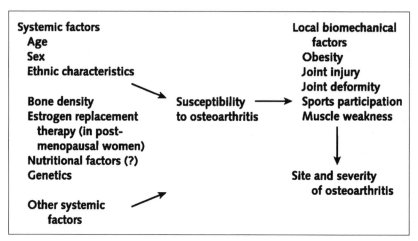

Systemic factors
  Age
  Sex
  Ethnic characteristics

  Bone density
  Estrogen replacement
    therapy (in post-
    menopausal women)
  Nutritional factors (?)
  Genetics

  Other systemic
    factors

Susceptibility → to osteoarthritis

Local biomechanical factors
Obesity
Joint injury
Joint deformity
Sports participation
Muscle weakness

Site and severity of osteoarthritis

Fig. 2. Pathogenesis of OA with putative risk factors. (*Adapted from* Dieppe P. The classification and diagnosis of osteoarthritis. In: Kuettner K, Goldberg V, eds. Osteoarthritic Disorders. Rosemont, IL: American Academy of Orthopaedic Surgeons; 1995; with permission.)

investigations to hypothesize that hormonal factors may play a role in the development of OA. However, results on effect of estrogen, either endogenous or exogenous, on OA from observational studies have been conflicting.[17–19] In a randomized clinical trial (the Heart and Estrogen/Progestin Replacement Study) in a group of older postmenopausal women with heart disease, no significant difference was found in the prevalence of knee pain or its associated disability between those taking estrogen plus progestin therapy or those taking placebo.[20] Data from the Women's Health Initiative showed that women on estrogen replacement therapy were 15% less likely to require total knee or hip arthroplasty than those not taking such therapy (hazard ratio 0.86; 95% confidence interval 0.70–1.00), but that estrogen combined with progestin therapy was not associated with the risk of joint replacement.[21]

Race/Ethnicity

The prevalence of OA and patterns of joints affected by OA vary among racial and ethnic groups. Both hip and hand OA were much less frequent among Chinese in the Beijing Osteoarthritis Study than in whites in the Framingham Study,[22,23] but Chinese women in the Beijing Osteoarthritis Study had significantly higher prevalence of both radiographic and symptomatic knee OA than white women in the Framingham Study.[24] Results from the Johnston County Osteoarthritis Project have shown that the prevalence of hip OA in African American women (23%) was similar to that in white women (22%), and prevalence was slightly higher in African American men (21%) than that in white men (17%).[25] It is of interest that prevalence of individual radiographic features of hip OA varied between African Americans compared with whites. For example, superior joint space narrowing and osteophytes at lateral compartment are more common in African Americans than in whites.[25] In addition, African Americans were also more likely to have more severe and tricompartmental osteophytes than their white counterparts.[26] Whether some of these racial/ethnic differences are related to differences in anatomic femoral and acetabular features, shown to be important in radiographic hip OA in whites,[27,28] is worthy of further study.

Genetics

Results from several studies have shown that OA is inherited and may vary by joint site. Twin and family studies have estimated the heritable component of OA to be between 50% and 65% with larger genetic influences for hand and hip OA than for knee OA.[29–31] In a genome-wide association study, Kerkhof and colleagues[32] reported that the C allele of rs3815148 on chromosome 7q22 was associated with a 1.14-fold increased prevalence of knee and/or hand OA and also with a 30% increased risk of knee OA progression. Several studies also found that an inverse association between general joint hypermobility, a lone benign trait, with hand and knee OA and serum cartilage oligometric matrix protein levels.[33,34]

Congenital/Developmental Conditions

A few congenital or developmental abnormalities (ie, congenital subluxation, Legg-Calvé-Perthes disease, and slipped capital femoral epiphysis) have been associated with occurrence of hip OA in later life[35–37]; however, because these developmental deformities are uncommon, they probably only account for a small proportion of the hip OA in the general population. Several studies have examined subclinical acetabular dysplasia, a more common, milder developmental abnormality, in relation to hip OA, with conflicting results.[27,38–41] Lane and colleagues[27] reported that abnormal center-edge angle or acetabular dysplasia were each associated with an approximately three-fold increased risk of incident hip OA in women,[27] suggesting that subclinical acetabular dysplasia may be a significant risk factor for the development of hip OA.

Diet

Dietary factors are the subject of considerable interest in OA; results of studies, however, are conflicting. One of the most promising nutritional factors for OA is vitamin D. Without sufficient vitamin D, bones can become thin, brittle, or misshapen. In the Framingham Study subjects in the lowest (<27 ng/mL) and middle (27.0–33.0 ng/mL) tertile of serum 25-hydroxyvitamin D had a threefold increased risk for progressive knee OA compared with those in the highest tertile; however, no such effect was observed for risk of incident disease.[42] In the Study of Osteoporotic Fractures, women in the middle (23–29 ng/mL) and lowest (8–22 ng/mL) tertiles of serum 25-vitamin D were 3 times as likely to develop incident hip OA, defined by joint space narrowing, as those in the highest tertile (30–72 ng/mL). However, serum vitamin D levels were not associated with the risk of hip OA characterized by osteophytes or with new disease defined according to the summary grade.[43] However, results from 2 cohort studies failed to confirm any protective effect of vitamin D on the structural worsening of knee OA.[44] A randomized, placebo-controlled clinical trial of vitamin D is currently underway to examine whether this vitamin can affect knee symptoms and cartilage loss measured on MRI in established knee OA.

Low vitamin C dietary intake was associated with an increased risk of progression, but not incidence, of both radiographic and symptomatic knee OA among the participants in the Framingham Study.[45] In the Johnston County Osteoarthritis Project subjects with a high ratio of $\alpha:\gamma$ tocopherol had 50% lower risk in development of radiographic knee OA.[46] However, results from a controlled clinical trial of vitamin E failed to ameliorate symptoms in patients who had symptomatic knee OA or to prevent knee OA progression, as measured by cartilage volume by MRI.[47]

Animal studies have shown that selenium deficiency is associated with irregular bone formation, decreased bone strength, and abnormalities in type I and II collage in cartilage.[48,49] In areas of China and eastern Asian where selenium levels in the soil are extremely low, the prevalence of Kashin-Beck disease, an early onset of osteoarthropathy, was also high and food supplementation with selenium decreased the incidence of this disease.[50,51] Preliminary results from the Johnston County Osteoarthritis Project have shown that suboptimal selenium levels, measured in toenails, were associated with worse knee OA.[52] However, others have reported that high selenium intake was significantly associated with increased risk of both hip and knee OA.[53]

In one study, high levels of serum vitamin K were associated with a low prevalence of radiographic hand OA, particularly for the presence of large osteophytes.[54] The relation of serum vitamin K levels to knee radiographic OA is less clear. A recent randomized, placebo-controlled trial of vitamin K supplementation (phylloquinone, 500 µg/d) did not confirm a protective effect of vitamin K on the severity of radiographic hand OA.

LOCAL RISK FACTORS
Obesity

Obesity and overweight have long been recognized as potent risk factors for OA, especially OA of the knee.[1] The results from the Framingham Study demonstrated that women who had lost about 5 kg had a 50% reduction in the risk of development of symptomatic knee OA.[55] The same study also found that weight loss was strongly associated with a reduced risk of development of radiographic knee OA. Weight-loss interventions have been shown to decrease pain and disability in established knee OA.[56,57] The Arthritis, Diet, and Activity Promotion Trial showed that weight loss combined with exercise, but neither weight loss nor exercise alone, were effective in decreasing pain and improving function in obese elders who had symptomatic knee OA.[56] Results from a meta-analysis concluded that although the effects of weight loss on pain were less consistent, weight reduction by about 5% was associated with an improvement of physical function.[57]

The relationship between overweight and hip OA is inconsistent and, if it exists, is weaker than that with knee OA.[58,59] There is, however, more consistent evidence that obesity increases the risk of bilateral radiographic as well as symptomatic hip OA.[60] In the Nurses' Health Study, higher BMI, especially BMI at age 18, was strongly associated with an increased risk of total hip replacement therapy.[61] Increased loading on the joint is probably the main, but not only, mechanism by which obesity causes knee or hip OA. Overloading the knee and hip joints could lead to synovial joint breakdown and failure of ligamentous and other structural support.

Injury/Surgery

Numerous studies have shown that knee injury is one of the strongest risk factors for OA. Severe injury to the structures of a joint, particularly a transarticular fracture, meniscal tear requiring meniscectomy, or anterior cruciate ligament injury, can result in an increased risk of OA development and musculoskeletal symptomatology.[62,63] In the Framingham Study the prevalence of meniscal damage was much higher among subjects with radiographic knee OA (82%) than those without OA (25%). The prevalence of meniscal damage increased with an increase in K/L grade ($P<.001$ for trend); among those with moderate (K/L = 3) and severe (K/L = 4) radiographic knee OA, 95% had evidence of meniscal damage.[64]

OCCUPATION

Repetitive use of joints at work is associated with an increased risk of OA. Studies have found that farmers have a high prevalence of hip OA.[65] The prevalence of

Heberden nodes was much higher in cotton mill workers, whereas spinal OA was no more common in these workers than in controls.[66] Workers whose jobs required repeated pincer grip had more OA at distal interphalangeal joints than did workers whose job required power grip.[67]

The risk of development of knee OA was more than 2 times greater for men whose jobs required both carrying and kneeling or squatting in mid-life than for those whose jobs did not require these physical activities.[68] The risks of knee OA associated with kneeling and squatting were much higher among subjects who were overweight or whose job also involved lifting.[69]

Physical Activity/Sports

Studies examining the relationship between sports activities and subsequent OA have produced conflicting results. There is some evidence that elite long-distance runners are at high risk for the development of knee and hip OA,[70-72] and that elite soccer players are at higher risk of getting knee OA compared with athletes who do not play soccer.[71,73] Surprisingly, the general level of physical activity itself may also increase the risk of OA. For instance, physical activity among elderly subjects in the Framingham Study was generally characterized by leisure-time walking and gardening. However, persons who engaged in relatively high levels of such activity had a threefold greater risk of developing radiographic knee OA than sedentary persons over 8 years of follow-up.[74] Similar findings were reported in another study in which women who had a high lifetime level of physical activity had a high prevalence of hip OA.[75] By contrast, others have shown that, in the absence of acute injury, recreational (moderate) long-distance running and jogging did not appear to increase the risk of OA.[76,77]

Mechanical Factors

The relationship between muscle strength and OA is complex, may vary by joint site, and is not entirely understood. Muscle weakness and atrophy commonly associated with knee OA had been thought to be the product of disuse resulting from pain avoidance. One study reported that women who had asymptomatic radiographic knee OA but had no muscle atrophy showed quadriceps muscle weakness,[78] suggesting that this might be a risk factor for the development of symptomatic knee OA.[78] Baker and colleagues[79] confirmed that persons who had both asymptomatic patellofemoral and tibiofemoral radiographic knee OA had weaker quadriceps strength than those who did not have OA.[79] In a follow-up study quadriceps muscle weakness not only resulted from painful knee OA but also increased the risk of knee structural damage.[80,81] Other studies,[82] however, showed that greater quadriceps muscle strength in the setting of malalignment and laxity may actually be associated with an increased risk of knee OA progression.

Using the data from the Genetics of Generalized Osteoarthritis Study, Dominick and colleagues[83] found an inverse cross-sectional association between grip strength and OA of the carpometacarpal joint and between pinch strength and OA of the metacarpophalangeal joint. On the other hand, greater grip strength was associated with an increased risk of radiographic hand OA among the participants of the Framingham Study: men whose maximal grip strength was in the highest tertile had a threefold increased risk of OA in the proximal interphalangeal, metacarpophalangeal, or thumb base joints, as compared with those with lowest tertile.[84] The investigators suggested that the maximal force exerted on specific joints might influence development of OA in those joints.

Alignment

Knee alignment (ie, the hip-knee-ankle angle) is a key determinant of load distribution. Any shift from a neutral or collinear alignment of the hip, knee, and ankle affects load distribution at the knee. Therefore, one would speculate that malaligned knees may have a higher risk of developing OA and a higher subsequent risk of progression than knees with neutral alignment.

In a prospective cohort study, Sharma and colleagues[85] demonstrated that in the presence of existing knee OA, abnormal anatomic alignment was strongly associated with accelerated structural deterioration in the compartment under greatest compressive stress.[85] Knees with varus alignment at baseline had a fourfold increase in the risk of medial progression of knee OA, and those with valgus alignment at baseline had a nearly fivefold increase in the risk of lateral progression. The same study also found that the impact of varus or valgus malalignment on the risk of OA progression was greater in knees with more severe baseline radiographic disease than knees with mild or moderate disease.[86] Another study found that knee malalignment was associated with the size and progression of bone marrow lesions as well as with rapid cartilage loss on MRI.[87]

The association between malalignment and risk of incident knee OA is less clear, however. The results from the Rotterdam study found that among knees with K/L grade 0 and 1, knees with valgus alignment had a 54% increased risk and knees with varus alignment had a twofold increased risk for the development of radiographic knee OA, compared with normal aligned knees.[88] In the Framingham Study, however, Hunter and colleagues,[89] using 4 measures of knee joint alignment (ie, the anatomic axis, the condylar angle, the tibial plateau angle, and the condylar tibial plateau angle), found none of these measures to be associated with an increased risk of incident radiographic knee OA. The investigators speculated that malalignment may not be a primary risk factor for the occurrence of radiographic knee OA but rather a marker of disease severity and/or its progression.

Laxity

Knee laxity is another potential risk factor for knee OA. Varus-valgus knee laxity is greater in the nonarthritic knees of patients who have idiopathic disease than in the knees of controls, suggesting that a portion of the increased laxity of knee OA precedes disease development and may predispose to disease.[90] Moreover, sagittal plane or anterior-posterior laxity may be increased in persons who have mild OA, and anterior-posterior laxity seems to decline with increasing severity of knee OA.[91,92] Because knee laxity may be altered by the disease itself, longitudinal data will be helpful in confirming these relationships.

Another factor that can alter biomechanics at the knee and hip is limb length inequality (LLI). In the Johnston County Osteoarthritis Project persons with an LLI of at least 2 cm were almost twice as likely to have radiographic knee OA and 40% more likely to have knee symptoms.[93] The results from the Multicenter Osteoarthritis Study also demonstrated that leg length inequality of 1 cm or more was not only associated with a higher prevalence of prevalent radiographic knee OA but also increased the risk of incident symptomatic and progressive knee OA.[94] These results point to LLI as a potentially modifiable risk factor for knee OA.

RISK FACTORS FOR SYMPTOMATIC OSTEOARTHRITIS

Although symptomatic knee OA is common, causes substantial disability, and consumes tremendous medical costs, most previous studies have focused on risk factors for radiographic OA.[1] Not all risk factors for radiographic OA are strong predictors of joint symptoms.[1,15] Women with radiographic knee OA were more likely to have symptoms than men,[95] and African Americans generally reported more knee and hip symptoms than whites.[96] Strenuous physical activity, especially activities requiring kneeling, knee-bending, squatting, and prolonged standing,[74,97] as well as knee injury and trauma,[98] have also been linked to a high prevalence of symptomatic knee OA. People who have severe radiographic OA are more likely to report joint pain than those with milder radiographic abnormalities.[9] Results from 2 observational studies[99] have demonstrated that there was a strong dose-response relation of the severity of radiographic knee OA to the prevalence of frequent knee pain, consistent frequent knee pain, and pain severity. Furthermore, joint space narrowing was more strongly associated with each pain measure than were osteophytes.

A few studies have demonstrated that several morphologic and pathologic changes detected by MRI, namely bone marrow lesions,[100,101] synovitis,[102,103] effusion,[102] or periarticular lesions[104] in the knee, were associated with knee pain, but others have failed to confirm the association between bone marrow lesions and knee pain.[105]

Studying risk factors for symptomatic OA is challenging. While pain in OA has long been considered chronic, it is not necessarily constant. Physicians often notice that clinically, patients with OA experience episodes of recurrent pain or pain exacerbation over the course of the disease. The pain from OA often worsens by using the involved joints, and lessens or is relieved with rest. Such pain patterns are also observed in epidemiologic studies. Gooberman-Hill and colleagues[106] reported that joint pain among subjects with knee or hip OA is often intermittent and variable, and adaptation and avoidance strategies modify the experience of pain. Because of methodological and logistical difficulties, however, few studies have been conducted to examine the dynamic relationship between risk factors and pain fluctuation. One such study used weekly telephone interviews over 12 weeks to assess the impact of fluctuations in knee or hip pain. Fluctuations were frequent and were observed in about 49% of individuals, and decreases in pain were associated with improved function, decreased work absenteeism, sleep disruption, and health care resource use.[107]

SUMMARY

Evolving definitions of OA and improvement in risk factor measurement, by using advanced imaging, systemic and local biomarkers, and improved methods for measuring symptoms and their impact, can help to elucidate mechanisms and identify potential areas for intervention or prevention. The application of these new sources of knowledge about the OA process holds promise for the development of new, potentially disease-modifying pharmaceuticals and nonpharmacologic therapies.

REFERENCES

1. Felson DT, Lawrence RC, Dieppe PA, et al. Osteoarthritis: new insights. Part 1: the disease and its risk factors. Ann Intern Med 2000;133(8):635–46.
2. Arthritis and Joint Pain. In: The Burden of Musculoskeletal Diseases in the United States. p. 71–96, Chapter 4. Available at: http://www.boneandjointburden.org. Accessed May 1, 2010.
3. Hadler NM. Knee pain is the malady—not osteoarthritis. Ann Intern Med 1992; 116(7):598–9.
4. Guccione AA, Felson DT, Anderson JJ, et al. The effects of specific medical conditions on the functional limitations of elders in the Framingham Study. Am J Public Health 1994;84(3):351–8.
5. DeFrances CJ, Podgornik MN. 2004 National Hospital Discharge Survey. Adv Data 2006;371:1–19.

6. Lawrence RC, Felson DT, Helmick CG, et al. Estimates of the prevalence of arthritis and other rheumatic conditions in the United States. Part II. Arthritis Rheum 2008;58(1):26–35.
7. Kellgren J, Lawrence JIn: Atlas of standard radiographs. The epidemiology of chronic rheumatism, vol. 2. Oxford (UK): Blackwell Scientific Publications; 1963.
8. Altman RD, Bloch DA, Dougados M, et al. Measurement of structural progression in osteoarthritis of the hip: the Barcelona consensus group. Osteoarthritis Cartilage 2004;12(7):515–24.
9. Brandt KD, Mazzuca SA, Conrozier T, et al. Which is the best radiographic protocol for a clinical trial of a structure modifying drug in patients with knee osteoarthritis? J Rheumatol 2002;29(6):1308–20.
10. Hernborg JS, Nilsson BE. The natural course of untreated osteoarthritis of the knee. Clin Orthop 1977;123:130–7.
11. Ahlback S. Osteoarthrosis of the knee. A radiographic investigation. Acta Radiol Diagn (Stockh) 1968;277(Suppl):7–72.
12. Hannan MT, Felson DT, Pincus T. Analysis of the discordance between radiographic changes and knee pain in osteoarthritis of the knee. J Rheumatol 2000;27(6):1513–7.
13. Oliveria SA, Felson DT, Reed JI, et al. Incidence of symptomatic hand, hip, and knee osteoarthritis among patients in a health maintenance organization. Arthritis Rheum 1995;38(8):1134–41.
14. Murphy L, Schwartz TA, Helmick CG, et al. Lifetime risk of symptomatic knee osteoarthritis. Arthritis Rheum 2008;59(9):1207–13.
15. Felson DT, Zhang Y. An update on the epidemiology of knee and hip osteoarthritis with a view to prevention. Arthritis Rheum 1998;41(8):1343–55.
16. Srikanth VK, Fryer JL, Zhai G, et al. A meta-analysis of sex differences prevalence, incidence and severity of osteoarthritis. Osteoarthritis Cartilage 2005;13(9):769–81.
17. Wluka AE, Cicuttini FM, Spector TD. Menopause, oestrogens and arthritis. Maturitas 2000;35(3):183–99.
18. Hannan MT, Felson DT, Anderson JJ, et al. Estrogen use and radiographic osteoarthritis of the knee in women. The Framingham Osteoarthritis Study. Arthritis Rheum 1990;33(4):525–32.
19. Nevitt MC, Cummings SR, Lane NE, et al. Association of estrogen replacement therapy with the risk of osteoarthritis of the hip in elderly white women. Study of Osteoporotic Fractures Research Group. Arch Intern Med 1996;156(18):2073–80.
20. Nevitt MC, Felson DT, Williams EN, et al. The effect of estrogen plus progestin on knee symptoms and related disability in postmenopausal women: The Heart and Estrogen/Progestin Replacement Study, a randomized, double-blind, placebo-controlled trial. Arthritis Rheum 2001;44(4):811–8.
21. Cirillo DJ, Wallace RB, Wu L, et al. Effect of hormone therapy on risk of hip and knee joint replacement in the Women's Health Initiative. Arthritis Rheum 2006;54(10):3194–204.
22. Nevitt MC, Xu L, Zhang YQ, et al. Very low prevalence of hip osteoarthritis among Chinese elderly in Beijing compared to Caucasians in the U.S.: the Beijing Osteoarthritis Study. Arthritis Rheum 2002;46(7):1773–9.
23. Zhang YQ, Xu L, Nevitt MC, et al. Chinese have a much lower prevalence of radiographic osteoarthritis of the hand than Caucasians in the U.S. Arthritis Rheum 2001;44(9):s225.

24. Zhang Y, Xu L, Nevitt MC, et al. Comparison of the prevalence of knee osteoarthritis between the elderly Chinese population in Beijing and whites in the United States: the Beijing Osteoarthritis Study. Arthritis Rheum 2001;44(9):2065–71.
25. Nelson E, Braga L, Benner J, et al. Characterization of individual radiographic features of hip osteoarthritis in African American and White women and men: the Johnston County Osteoarthritis Project. Arthritis Care Res (Hoboken) 2010;62(2):190–7.
26. Braga L, Renner JB, Schwartz TA, et al. Differences in radiographic features of knee osteoarthritis in African-Americans and Caucasians: the Johnston County Osteoarthritis Project. Osteoarthritis Cartilage 2009;17(12):1554–61.
27. Lane NE, Lin P, Christiansen L, et al. Association of mild acetabular dysplasia with an increased risk of incident hip osteoarthritis in elderly white women: the study of osteoporotic fractures. Arthritis Rheum 2000;43(2):400–4.
28. Lynch JA, Parimi N, Chaganti RK, et al. The association of proximal femoral shape and incident radiographic hip OA in elderly women. Osteoarthritis Cartilage 2009;17(10):1313–8.
29. Spector TD, Cicuttini F, Baker J, et al. Genetic influences on osteoarthritis in women: a twin study. BMJ 1996;312(7036):940–3.
30. Palotie A, Vaisanen P, Ott J, et al. Predisposition to familial osteoarthrosis linked to type II collagen gene. Lancet 1989;1(8644):924–7.
31. Felson DT, Couropmitree NN, Chaisson CE, et al. Evidence for a Mendelian gene in a segregation analysis of generalized radiographic osteoarthritis: the Framingham Study. Arthritis Rheum 1998;41(6):1064–71.
32. Kerkhof HJ, Lories RJ, Meulenbelt I, et al. A genome-wide association study identifies an osteoarthritis susceptibility locus on chromosome 7q22. Arthritis Rheum 2010;62(2):499–510.
33. Dolan AL, Hart DJ, Doyle DV, et al. The relationship of joint hypermobility, bone mineral density, and osteoarthritis in the general population: the Chingford Study. J Rheumatol 2003;30(4):799–803.
34. Chen HC, Shah SH, Li YJ, et al. Inverse association of general joint hypermobility with hand and knee osteoarthritis and serum cartilage oligomeric matrix protein levels. Arthritis Rheum 2008;58(12):3854–64.
35. Murray RO. The aetiology of primary osteoarthritis of the hip. Br J Radiol 1965; 38(455):810–24.
36. Stulberg SD, Cooperman DR, Wallensten R. The natural history of Legg-Calve-Perthes disease. J Bone Joint Surg Am 1981;63(7):1095–108.
37. Harris WH. Etiology of osteoarthritis of the hip. Clin Orthop Relat Res 1986;213: 20–33.
38. Croft P, Cooper C, Wickham C, et al. Osteoarthritis of the hip and acetabular dysplasia. Ann Rheum Dis 1991;50(5):308–10.
39. Smith RW, Egger P, Coggon D, et al. Osteoarthritis of the hip joint and acetabular dysplasia in women. Ann Rheum Dis 1995;54(3):179–81.
40. Lau EM, Lin F, Lam D, et al. Hip osteoarthritis and dysplasia in Chinese men. Ann Rheum Dis 1995;54(12):965–9.
41. Lane NE, Nevitt MC, Cooper C, et al. Acetabular dysplasia and osteoarthritis of the hip in elderly white women. Ann Rheum Dis 1997;56(10):627–30.
42. McAlindon TE, Felson DT, Zhang Y, et al. Relation of dietary intake and serum levels of vitamin D to progression of osteoarthritis of the knee among participants in the Framingham Study. Ann Intern Med 1996;125(5):353–9.
43. Lane NE, Gore LR, Cummings SR, et al. Serum vitamin D levels and incident changes of radiographic hip osteoarthritis: a longitudinal study. Study

of Osteoporotic Fractures Research Group. Arthritis Rheum 1999;42(5): 854–60.

44. Felson DT, Niu J, Clancy M, et al. Low levels of vitamin D and worsening of knee osteoarthritis: results of two longitudinal studies. Arthritis Rheum 2007;56(1): 129–36.

45. McAlindon TE, Jacques P, Zhang Y, et al. Do antioxidant micronutrients protect against the development and progression of knee osteoarthritis? Arthritis Rheum 1996;39(4):648–56.

46. Jordan JM, De Roos AJ, Renner JB, et al. A case-control study of serum tocopherol levels and the alpha- to gamma-tocopherol ratio in radiographic knee osteoarthritis: the Johnston County Osteoarthritis Project. Am J Epidemiol 2004; 159(10):968–77.

47. Wluka AE, Stuckey S, Brand C, et al. Supplementary vitamin E does not affect the loss of cartilage volume in knee osteoarthritis: a 2 year double blind randomized placebo controlled study. J Rheumatol 2002;29(12):2585–91.

48. Sasaki S, Iwata H, Ishiguro N, et al. Low-selenium diet, bone, and articular cartilage in rats. Nutrition 1994;10(6):538–43.

49. Turan B, Balcik C, Akkas N. Effect of dietary selenium and vitamin E on the biomechanical properties of rabbit bones. Clin Rheumatol 1997;16(5):441–9.

50. Fang W, Wu P, Hu R, et al. Environmental Se-Mo-B deficiency and its possible effects on crops and Keshan-Beck disease (KBD) in the Chousang area, Yao County, Shaanxi Province, China. Environ Geochem Health 2003;25(2):267–80.

51. Moreno-Reyes R, Mathieu F, Boelaert M, et al. Selenium and iodine supplementation of rural Tibetan children affected by Kashin-Beck osteoarthropathy. Am J Clin Nutr 2003;78(1):137–44.

52. Jordan JM, Fang F, Arab L, et al. Low selenium levels are associated with increased risk for osteoarthritis of the knee. Arthritis Rheum 2005;52:s455.

53. Engstrom G, De Verdier MG, Nilsson PM, et al. Incidence of severe knee and hip osteoarthritis in relation to dietary intake of antioxidants beta-carotene, vitamin C, vitamin E and selenium: a population-based prospective cohort study. Arthritis Rheum 2009;60:s235–6.

54. Neogi T, Booth SL, Zhang YQ, et al. Low vitamin K status is associated with osteoarthritis in the hand and knee. Arthritis Rheum 2006;54(4):1255–61.

55. Felson DT, Zhang Y, Anthony JM, et al. Weight loss reduces the risk for symptomatic knee osteoarthritis in women. The Framingham Study. Ann Intern Med 1992;116(7):535–9.

56. Messier SP, Loeser RF, Miller GD, et al. Exercise and dietary weight loss in overweight and obese older adults with knee osteoarthritis: the Arthritis, Diet, and Activity Promotion Trial. Arthritis Rheum 2004;50(5):1501–10.

57. Christensen R, Bartels EM, Astrup A, et al. Effect of weight reduction in obese patients diagnosed with knee osteoarthritis: a systematic review and meta-analysis. Ann Rheum Dis 2007;66(4):433–9.

58. Tepper S, Hochberg MC. Factors associated with hip osteoarthritis: data from the First National Health and Nutrition Examination Survey (NHANES-I). Am J Epidemiol 1993;137(10):1081–8.

59. van Saase JL, Vandenbroucke JP, van Romunde LK, et al. Osteoarthritis and obesity in the general population. A relationship calling for an explanation. J Rheumatol 1988;15(7):1152–8.

60. Heliovaara M, Makela M, Impivaara O, et al. Association of overweight, trauma and workload with coxarthrosis. A health survey of 7,217 persons. Acta Orthop Scand 1993;64(5):513–8.

61. Karlson EW, Mandl LA, Aweh GN, et al. Total hip replacement due to osteoarthritis: the importance of age, obesity, and other modifiable risk factors. Am J Med 2003;114(2):93–8.
62. Lohmander LS, Ostenberg A, Englund M, et al. High prevalence of knee osteoarthritis, pain, and functional limitations in female soccer players twelve years after anterior cruciate ligament injury. Arthritis Rheum 2004;50(10):3145–52.
63. Roos EM, Ostenberg A, Roos H, et al. Long-term outcome of meniscectomy: symptoms, function, and performance tests in patients with or without radiographic osteoarthritis compared to matched controls. Osteoarthritis Cartilage 2001;9(4):316–24.
64. Englund M, Guermazi A, Gale D, et al. Incidental meniscal findings on knee MRI in middle-aged and elderly persons. N Engl J Med 2008;359(11):1108–15.
65. Croft P, Cooper C, Wickham C, et al. Osteoarthritis of the hip and occupational activity. Scand J Work Environ Health 1992;18(1):59–63.
66. Lawrence JS. Rheumatism in cotton operatives. Br J Ind Med 1961;18:270–6.
67. Hadler NM, Gillings DB, Imbus HR, et al. Hand structure and function in an industrial setting. Arthritis Rheum 1978;21(2):210–20.
68. Felson DT, Hannan MT, Naimark A, et al. Occupational physical demands, knee bending, and knee osteoarthritis: results from the Framingham Study. J Rheumatol 1991;18(10):1587–92.
69. Coggon D, Croft P, Kellingray S, et al. Occupational physical activities and osteoarthritis of the knee. Arthritis Rheum 2000;43(7):1443–9.
70. Puranen J, Ala-Ketola L, Peltokallio P, et al. Running and primary osteoarthritis of the hip. Br Med J 1975;2(5968):424–5.
71. Kujala UM, Kettunen J, Paananen H, et al. Knee osteoarthritis in former runners, soccer players, weight lifters, and shooters. Arthritis Rheum 1995;38(4):539–46.
72. Spector TD, Harris PA, Hart DJ, et al. Risk of osteoarthritis associated with long-term weight-bearing sports: a radiologic survey of the hips and knees in female ex-athletes and population controls. Arthritis Rheum 1996;39(6):988–95.
73. Roos H, Lindberg H, Gardsell P, et al. The prevalence of gonarthrosis and its relation to meniscectomy in former soccer players. Am J Sports Med 1994; 22(2):219–22.
74. McAlindon TE, Wilson PW, Aliabadi P, et al. Level of physical activity and the risk of radiographic and symptomatic knee osteoarthritis in the elderly: the Framingham Study. Am J Med 1999;106(2):151–7.
75. Lane NE, Hochberg MC, Pressman A, et al. Recreational physical activity and the risk of osteoarthritis of the hip in elderly women. J Rheumatol 1999;26(4): 849–54.
76. Lane NE, Michel B, Bjorkengren A, et al. The risk of osteoarthritis with running and aging: a 5-year longitudinal study. J Rheumatol 1993;20(3):461–8.
77. Newton PM, Mow VC, Gardner TR, et al. Winner of the 1996 Cabaud Award. The effect of lifelong exercise on canine articular cartilage. Am J Sports Med 1997; 25(3):282–7.
78. Slemenda C, Brandt KD, Heilman DK, et al. Quadriceps weakness and osteoarthritis of the knee. Ann Intern Med 1997;127(2):97–104.
79. Baker KR, Xu L, Zhang Y, et al. Quadriceps weakness and its relationship to tibiofemoral and patellofemoral knee osteoarthritis in Chinese: the Beijing Osteoarthritis Study. Arthritis Rheum 2004;50(6):1815–21.
80. Slemenda C, Heilman DK, Brandt KD, et al. Reduced quadriceps strength relative to body weight: a risk factor for knee osteoarthritis in women? Arthritis Rheum 1998;41(11):1951–9.

81. Brandt KD, Heilman DK, Slemenda C, et al. Quadriceps strength in women with radiographically progressive osteoarthritis of the knee and those with stable radiographic changes. J Rheumatol 1999;26(11):2431–7.
82. Sharma L, Dunlop DD, Cahue S, et al. Quadriceps strength and osteoarthritis progression in malaligned and lax knees. Ann Intern Med 2003;138(8):613–9.
83. Dominick KL, Jordan JM, Renner JB, et al. Relationship of radiographic and clinical variables to pinch and grip strength among individuals with osteoarthritis. Arthritis Rheum 2005;52(5):1424–30.
84. Chaisson CE, Zhang Y, Sharma L, et al. Grip strength and the risk of developing radiographic hand osteoarthritis: results from the Framingham Study. Arthritis Rheum 1999;42(1):33–8.
85. Sharma L, Song J, Felson DT, et al. The role of knee alignment in disease progression and functional decline in knee osteoarthritis. JAMA 2001;286(2):188–95.
86. Cerejo R, Dunlop DD, Cahue S, et al. The influence of alignment on risk of knee osteoarthritis progression according to baseline stage of disease. Arthritis Rheum 2002;46(10):2632–6.
87. Felson DT, McLaughlin S, Goggins J, et al. Bone marrow edema and its relation to progression of knee osteoarthritis. Ann Intern Med 2003;139(5 Pt 1):330–6.
88. Brouwer GM, van Tol AW, Bergink AP, et al. Association between valgus and varus alignment and the development and progression of radiographic osteoarthritis of the knee. Arthritis Rheum 2007;56(4):1204–11.
89. Hunter DJ, Niu J, Felson DT, et al. Knee alignment does not predict incident osteoarthritis: the Framingham Osteoarthritis Study. Arthritis Rheum 2007;56(4):1212–8.
90. Sharma L, Lou C, Felson DT, et al. Laxity in healthy and osteoarthritic knees. Arthritis Rheum 1999;42(5):861–70.
91. Wada M, Imura S, Baba H, et al. Knee laxity in patients with osteoarthritis and rheumatoid arthritis. Br J Rheumatol 1996;35(6):560–3.
92. Brage ME, Draganich LF, Pottenger LA, et al. Knee laxity in symptomatic osteoarthritis. Clin Orthop 1994;304:184–9.
93. Golightly YM, Allen KD, Renner JB, et al. Relationship of limb length inequality with radiographic knee and hip osteoarthritis. Osteoarthritis Cartilage 2007;15(7):824–9.
94. Harvey WF, Yang M, Cooke TD, et al. Association of leg-length inequality with knee osteoarthritis: a cohort study. Ann Intern Med 2010;152:287–95.
95. Felson DT, Naimark A, Anderson J, et al. The prevalence of knee osteoarthritis in the elderly. The Framingham Osteoarthritis Study. Arthritis Rheum 1987;30(8):914–8.
96. Jordan JM, Helmick CG, Renner JB, et al. Prevalence of knee symptoms and radiographic and symptomatic knee osteoarthritis in African Americans and Caucasians: the Johnston County Osteoarthritis Project. J Rheumatol 2007;34(1):172–80.
97. Maetzel A, Makela M, Hawker G, et al. Osteoarthritis of the hip and knee and mechanical occupational exposure—a systematic overview of the evidence. J Rheumatol 1997;24(8):1599–607.
98. Davis MA, Ettinger WH, Neuhaus JM, et al. The association of knee injury and obesity with unilateral and bilateral osteoarthritis of the knee. Am J Epidemiol 1989;130(2):278–88.
99. Neogi T, Felson D, Niu J, et al. Association between radiographic features of knee osteoarthritis and pain: results from two cohort studies. BMJ 2009;339:b2844.

100. Felson DT, Chaisson CE, Hill CL, et al. The association of bone marrow lesions with pain in knee osteoarthritis. Ann Intern Med 2001;134(7):541–9.
101. Felson DT, Niu J, Guermazi A, et al. Correlation of the development of knee pain with enlarging bone marrow lesions on magnetic resonance imaging. Arthritis Rheum 2007;56(9):2986–92.
102. Hill CL, Gale DG, Chaisson CE, et al. Knee effusions, popliteal cysts, and synovial thickening: association with knee pain in osteoarthritis. J Rheumatol 2001; 28(6):1330–7.
103. Hill CL, Hunter DJ, Niu J, et al. Synovitis detected on magnetic resonance imaging and its relation to pain and cartilage loss in knee osteoarthritis. Ann Rheum Dis 2007;66(12):1599–603.
104. Hill CL, Gale DR, Chaisson CE, et al. Periarticular lesions detected on magnetic resonance imaging: prevalence in knees with and without symptoms. Arthritis Rheum 2003;48(10):2836–44.
105. Link TM, Steinbach LS, Ghosh S, et al. Osteoarthritis: MR imaging findings in different stages of disease and correlation with clinical findings. Radiology 2003;226(2):373–81.
106. Gooberman-Hill R, Woolhead G, Mackichan F, et al. Assessing chronic joint pain: lessons from a Focus Group Study. Arthritis Rheum 2007;57(4):666–71.
107. Hutchings A, Calloway M, Choy E, et al. The Longitudinal Examination of Arthritis Pain (LEAP) Study: relationships between weekly fluctuations in patient-rated joint pain and other health outcomes. J Rheumatol 2007;34(11):2291–300.

Age-Related Changes in the Musculoskeletal System and the Development of Osteoarthritis

Richard F. Loeser, MD

KEYWORDS

- Aging • Osteoarthritis • Articular cartilage
- Elderly • Cell senescence • Oxidative stress

The prevalence of osteoarthritis (OA) increases with age such that 30% to 50% of adults older than 65 years suffer from this condition.[1,2] Radiographic changes of OA, in particular the presence of osteophytes, are even more common such that radiographic surveys of multiple joints (hands, spine, hips, and knees) reveal OA in at least one joint in over 80% of older adults.[3] However, only about half of people with radiographic OA experience significant symptoms. Likewise, not all older adults with symptoms of joint pain have radiographic evidence OA in the painful joint. In a study of 480 adults older than 65 years who reported chronic knee pain, only about 50% had radiographic evidence of knee OA.[4]

Although OA is most common in the hands, involvement of the knees and hips is usually much more disabling. Radiographic involvement of the distal interphalangeal joints in the hand was present in more than half of men older than 65 and more than half of women older than 55 years,[5] but only 13% of men and 26% of women older than 70 were found to have symptomatic hand OA.[6] The prevalence of radiographic knee osteoarthritis in subjects aged 60 years and older increased with each decade of life from 33% among those 60 to 70 years to 43.7% among those older

This work was supported by the National Institute on Aging (RO1 AG16697 and the Wake Forest University Claude D. Pepper Older Americans Independence Center P30 AG021332), the National Institute on Arthritis, Musculoskeletal and Skin Diseases (RO1 AR49003), the American Federation for Aging Research, and the Dorothy Rhyne Kimbrell and Willard Duke Kimbrell Professorship.
Section of Molecular Medicine, Wake Forest University School of Medicine, Medical Center Boulevard, Winston-Salem, NC 27157, USA
E-mail address: rloeser@wfubmc.edu

Clin Geriatr Med 26 (2010) 371–386
doi:10.1016/j.cger.2010.03.002
0749-0690/10/$ – see front matter

than 80 years, while the prevalence of symptomatic knee OA in these subjects was 9.5%, and increased with age in women but not men.[7] In the Johnson Country Osteoarthritis cohort, the prevalence of radiographic knee OA rose from 26.2% in the 55- to 64-year range to nearly half of participants in the 75+ group, and the prevalence of symptomatic knee OA likewise increased from 16.3% to 32.8% between these age groups.[8] Symptomatic hip OA in this cohort was reported as 5.9% in the 45- to 54-year age group, increasing to 17% in the 75+ age group.[9]

The relationship between aging and OA is well known but the mechanisms for how aging predisposes the joint to developing OA are still not fully understood. Changes intrinsic to the joint as well as those extrinsic (such as sarcopenia, altered bone remodeling, and reduced proprioception) contribute to the development of OA. The concept that aging contributes to, but does not directly cause OA, is consistent with the multifactorial nature of this condition and the disparity in which joints are most commonly affected. In this article, current concepts of the biology of OA are reviewed and the relationship between aging and the development of OA considered.

THE PATHOBIOLOGY OF OSTEOARTHRITIS

OA is a multifactorial condition, but the pathologic changes seen in osteoarthritic joints have common features no matter what the cause(s) of the condition in a given individual. These features include degradation of the articular cartilage starting at the joint surface and progressing to full thickness loss, thickening of the subchondral bone with accumulation of poorly mineralized matrix, osteophyte formation at the margins of joint surfaces, variable degrees of synovial inflammation with limited pannus formation, degeneration of ligaments and in the knee the menisci, with eventual ligamentous rupture and meniscal extrusion, and hypertrophy of the joint capsule contributing to joint enlargement (**Fig. 1**). In some individuals, increased subchondral bone remodeling results in bone marrow lesions detected on magnetic resonance imaging (MRI) and, in many older adults, calcification in the articular cartilage and/or the menisci is seen on plain radiographs. In the articular cartilage, the earliest changes at the joint surface occur in the areas that receive the greatest mechanical forces.

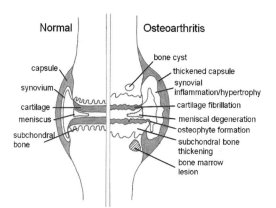

Fig. 1. Pathology of osteoarthritis. The osteoarthritic joint is characterized by degradation and loss of the articular cartilage, thickening of the subchondral bone accompanied by formation of bone marrow lesions and cysts, osteophytes at the joint margins, variable degrees of synovitis with synovial hypertrophy, meniscal degeneration (knee), and thickening of the joint capsule.

As OA progresses, the loss of the articular cartilage affects joint movement because of the loss of a smooth lubricated surface responsible for the normal gliding motion of the joint. The pathologic changes noted in the other joint tissues also contribute to the loss of normal joint function and, because unlike the cartilage they contain pain fibers, these tissues are responsible for the pain experienced by people with OA.

There are reasons to believe that although OA has common pathologic features seen once the disease becomes advanced, it may start with selected features that are dependent on the initiating factors in a given individual. For example, in an individual with posttraumatic OA resulting from rupture of the anterior cruciate ligament, the condition likely started with a period of acute joint inflammation with synovitis and cartilage matrix destruction followed later by development of bony changes, whereas in an individual with OA related to obesity it may have started with increased bone formation followed by articular cartilage matrix destruction and secondary synovial inflammation stimulated by release of cartilage matrix fragments. The early stages of OA have been difficult to study. Most people do not develop symptoms until significant joint damage has occurred, commonly after age 50 to 60 years, but there is radiographic evidence for OA in a significant percentage of women beginning in the early forties.[10] Researchers are attempting to develop biomarkers and advanced imaging techniques that could detect early-stage disease but, given the slowly progressive nature of OA, it will be some time before sufficient information is available to determine the predictive power of these techniques.

At the cell and tissue level, cartilage in OA is characterized by an imbalance in matrix synthesis and matrix degradation. The chondrocyte is the only cell type present in articular cartilage and therefore is responsible for both the synthesis and breakdown of the cartilaginous extracellular matrix.[11] Signals generated by cytokines, growth factors, and the matrix regulate chondrocyte metabolic activity. In the early stages of OA, there is evidence of increased matrix synthesis, although not all the matrix proteins produced are the same as those made by normal adult articular chondrocytes. There is increased expression of the fetal form of type II collagen (type IIA)[12] and of type III collagen and fibronectin,[13,14] as well as proteoglycans with altered sulfation patterns.[15] Excessive matrix degradation progressively overwhelms matrix synthesis, and this appears to be caused by inflammatory and catabolic signals that are present in excess of the anti-inflammatory and anabolic signals (**Fig. 2**). Proinflammatory cytokines found in OA cartilage include interleukin (IL)-1, IL-6, IL-7, IL-8, and tumor necrosis factor (TNF)-α, to name just a few. The presence of a large number of inflammatory mediators within the articular cartilage indicates that OA is much more inflammatory than previously thought. The excess of inflammatory signals inhibits matrix synthesis and promotes increased production of matrix degrading enzymes, including matrix metalloproteinases (MMPs), aggrecanases, and other proteases that degrade the cartilage matrix. As OA develops, chondrocytes can assume a hypertrophic phenotype characterized by production of type X collagen, alkaline phosphatase, and MMP-13 (collagenase-3).[13]

Chondrocyte death has been observed during the development of OA, but whether this is an early or late event is not clear.[16,17] Because cartilage lacks an abundant supply of stem or progenitor cells, the loss of chondrocytes to cell death results in a decline in cell numbers. This decline is most apparent in the superficial region of the articular cartilage. Although normally adult articular chondrocytes rarely divide, there is evidence for cell proliferation during the development of OA, resulting in clusters of chondrocytes being present. However, these cells are unable to maintain the matrix, which may be due at least in part to a reduced ability to respond to growth factor stimulation further contributing to an imbalance in matrix synthesis and degradation.

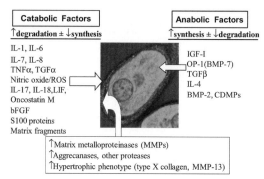

Catabolic Factors	Anabolic Factors
↑degradation ± ↓synthesis	↑synthesis ± ↓degradation
IL-1, IL-6	IGF-I
IL-7, IL-8	OP-1(BMP-7)
TNFα, TGFα	TGFβ
Nitric oxide/ROS	IL-4
IL-17, IL-18,LIF,	BMP-2, CDMPs
Oncostatin M	
bFGF	
S100 proteins	
Matrix fragments	

↑Matrix metalloproteinases (MMPs)
↑Aggrecanases, other proteases
↑Hypertrophic phenotype (type X collagen, MMP-13)

Fig. 2. Catabolic and anabolic factors that regulate chondrocyte function. A host of factors, produced locally by articular chondrocytes, regulate matrix synthesis and degradation in articular cartilage. As osteoarthritis develops, catabolic activators overwhelm anabolic factors resulting in an imbalance in matrix synthesis and degradation. Matrix degradation is mediated by MMPs, aggrecanase, and other proteases produced by the chondrocyte in response to the catabolic factors. A change in the chondrocyte phenotype to a hypertrophic phenotype also occurs, likely in response to one or more of the catabolic factors. BMP, bone morphogenetic protein; CDMP, cartilage-derived morphogenetic protein; FGF, fibroblast growth factor; IGF, insulin-like growth factor; IL, interleukin; OP, osteogenic protein; TGF, transforming growth factor; TNF, tumor necrosis factor.

In contrast to matrix loss in the articular cartilage, the subchondral bone undergoes increased matrix production, resulting in a thickening of this region. Older theories of OA suggested that the increased subchondral bone resulted in increased stiffness that contributed to the degradation of the overlying cartilage by increasing local stresses.[18,19] However, later studies found that the subchondral bone in OA was poorly mineralized and perhaps less stiff than normal bone.[18–20] More recently, studies have focused on inflammatory mediators produced by subchondral bone cells that could diffuse through the calcified cartilage zone or enter through cracks in the calcified cartilage to negatively affect the overlying articular cartilage.[21] The presence of localized areas of increased bone remodeling detected by bone scans or MRI has been noted in areas of cartilage loss, and is associated with pain in OA.[22] The correlation of these lesions in the knee with the location of excessive loading, that is, medial bone lesions in association with varus alignment and lateral lesions with valgus alignment, suggest they are mechanically mediated.[23]

The degree of synovitis present in OA is variable. In people with OA severe enough to require knee replacement, about one-third of patients had marked synovitis, one-third moderate synovitis, and one-third little to no synovitis,[24] which suggests that synovitis may be important in a subset of people with OA but that it is not required to progress to end-stage disease. However, an arthroscopic study of people with early OA did find an association between the presence of synovitis and progression of cartilage lesions measured a year later.[25] Studies of OA synovial fluid have revealed the presence of inflammatory cytokines that could be involved in stimulating cartilage destruction as well as destruction of other joint tissues such as the meniscus and ligaments. The growth factor transforming growth factor (TGF)-β, although an important contributor to cartilage matrix production, may be responsible for the stimulation of synovial hypertrophy as well as osteophyte formation.[26]

Although the synovium is involved in OA, the extent of inflammation is usually less than that found in rheumatoid arthritis (RA), where pannus formation is much more extensive and appears to be directly responsible for joint tissue destruction.

The extent of synovial inflammation as well as higher systemic levels of inflammatory mediators has been used to classify RA as inflammatory arthritis and OA as "noninflammatory." However, as noted earlier, inflammatory mediators are responsible for joint tissue destruction in OA and elevated serum levels of C-reactive protein,[27] and cytokines including IL-6[28] in people with OA indicate that inflammation plays a role in OA as well as RA.

RISK FACTORS FOR DEVELOPMENT OF OSTEOARTHRITIS IN THE ELDERLY

Besides age, the common risk factors for OA include obesity, previous joint injury, genetics, and anatomic factors including joint shape and alignment.[29] Additional factors include gender, race, and nutritional factors, such as vitamin D deficiency.[30,31] These risk factors appear to interact with age to determine which joints are affected by OA and how severe the condition will be (**Fig. 3**). A joint injury earlier in life predisposes that particular joint to OA later in life.[32] There is also evidence to suggest that an older adult will develop OA faster than a younger adult after an acute joint injury such as an anterior cruciate ligament tear.[33] Other age-related factors that contribute to the development of OA include a decline in muscle strength, loss of proprioception, degenerative changes in the meniscus and joint ligaments, increased bone turnover, and calcification of joint tissues.[29,34,35]

In terms of knee OA, recent MRI studies have revealed the important role of the meniscus. Incidental meniscal damage on MRI is quite common in the elderly, ranging from a prevalence of 19% in women aged 50 to 59 years to 56% in men in the 70- to 90-year-old age group.[36] The prevalence increased to 63% in symptomatic subjects with at least moderate radiographic OA measured by plain films. In a longitudinal study, symptomatic subjects with significant meniscal damage had an odds ratio of

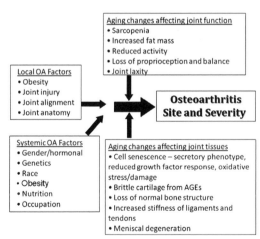

Fig. 3. Relationship between osteoarthritis risk factors and aging changes that interact to promote the development of osteoarthritis. OA is a multifactorial condition that is not simply the direct result of aging. Rather, aging changes increase the susceptibility to the development of OA when OA risk factors are also present. The OA factors are both local and systemic. Obesity can have local effects due to increased joint loading and systemic effects due to the production of adipokines and cytokines by adipose tissue that may contribute to the development of OA. The various aging and OA factors interact to influence the site and severity of the disease.

7.4 for the development of radiographic knee OA.[37] These studies suggest that age-related changes in the meniscus may contribute to meniscal degeneration that in turn may contribute to the development and progression of knee OA.

Recent MRI studies have also shown that anterior cruciate ligament (ACL) disruption is common in older adults with knee OA, even without a known history of trauma.[38] A well-known risk factor for the development of posttraumatic knee OA, age-related changes in the ACL may predispose the ligament to spontaneous rupture or rupture after minimal trauma. Changes that occur in aging ligaments such as increased stiffness from collagen cross-linking combined with decreasing fibril diameter may increase the risk for ACL tears.[39] Studies are needed to better characterize aging changes in joint ligaments and to determine if the mechanisms are similar to those occurring in other soft tissues in the joint such as the cartilage and meniscus.

As detailed earlier, the subchondral bone is clearly involved in the development of OA, and knowledge is being gained on the mechanisms that seem related to increased bone remodeling and the laying down of an abnormal matrix, processes that are potentially affected by aging.[19,40] Bone marrow lesions detected by MRI in people with OA are associated with pain and disease progression.[22,23,41] First thought to represent edema because of their bright appearance on T2-weighted MRI, these areas most likely represent areas of localized remodeling.[42] The association of bone marrow lesions with malalignment suggests excessive loading may play a role in their development. Increasing age has been shown to be a risk factor for the development of bone marrow lesions in asymptomatic individuals.[43] This is another area where future research may help elucidate how aging changes in a tissue outside of cartilage contributes to the risk of OA progression in older adults.

Finally, calcification and crystal formation within joint tissues are common findings in older adults that may play a role in OA progression. The association between calcium pyrophosphate deposition disease (CPPD) and the presence of radiographic osteoarthritis has been well established[35,44]; however, the role of calcium crystals in the progression of OA has been debated. Some believe that OA and CPPD are common but separate age-related conditions and others believe that the two are closely connected.[35,45,46] Because OA and calcium pyrophosphate are equally associated with osteophyte formation, it has been suggested that mechanical stress may induce release of chemokines that encourage both proliferative bone changes and calcium pyrophosphate formation.[47,48] Crystals within the articular cartilage or in the synovium could stimulate toll-like receptors on chondrocytes and synovial cells, resulting in production of inflammatory mediators.[49] Crystals may play a role in erosive OA, a more destructive form of OA seen most commonly in the distal digits of the hands in elderly women in which inflammation is a prominent component.[50,51]

THE CONTRIBUTION OF AGING IN CELLS AND TISSUES TO THE DEVELOPMENT OF OSTEOARTHRITIS
Cell Senescence

Most of the work to date on the relationship between aging changes at the cellular level and the development of OA has focused on the articular cartilage. Given the similarities between chondrocytes and meniscal cells these studies probably also relate to aging in the meniscus, but more studies need to be done in that specific tissue. Normally there is little to no cell turnover in adult articular cartilage[52] and so chondrocytes are thought to be long-lived cells and, as such, can accumulate age-related changes over many years. In many tissues, senescent cells can be replaced by differentiation of cells from a local pool of progenitor cells, but in adult articular cartilage it is not clear if such a pool exists. Recent studies have challenged the notion that cartilage does not contain progenitor cells, but these studies were performed with either bovine tissue from very young animals[53] or OA tissue,[54] the latter of which might have included cells from other tissues such as the synovium or bone marrow that can make their way to the cartilage when it is severely damaged. Even if there is a local pool of progenitor cells, they do not appear to be capable of replacing senescent, damaged, or dead cells in the articular cartilage.

There does appear to be an age-related reduction in the number of chondrocytes in cartilage and a further loss of cells in OA cartilage, but the extent of cell death is debated.[16,17,55] A 30% decrease in cell density between the ages of 30 and 70 years has been described in human hip specimens.[56] However, a study of human knees found less than 5% cell loss with aging.[52] Although many studies have reported apoptotic chondrocytes in OA cartilage,[17] few have examined apoptosis in cartilage with normal aging with the exception of a study in rat cartilage that found evidence of increased apoptosis with aging.[57] An age-related decline in levels of the high-mobility group box (HMGB) protein 2, which is expressed in the superficial zone of cartilage, might contribute to an increase in chondrocyte death.[58] HMGB2 is a nonhistone chromatin protein that can serve as a transcriptional regulator. Deletion of HMGB2 in transgenic mice was found to cause an early onset of OA-like changes in the superficial zone of cartilage that were associated with an increase in susceptibility of chondrocytes to cell death.

Chondrocytes have been shown to exhibit telomere shortening,[59] a classic feature of cell senescence, but because chondrocytes rarely divide it is unlikely that the shortened telomeres represent replicative senescence. Classic replicative senescence requires more than 30 to 40 population doublings,[60] which would be unlikely to occur in adult cartilage. Telomere shortening can also occur from extrinsic or "stress-induced" senescence that results from the chronic effects of oxidative damage, activated oncogenes, and inflammation.[61,62] This form of cell senescence is much more likely in cartilage, where oxidative stress and chronic inflammation could be factors.[63]

The concept of cell senescence has developed beyond classic replicative senescence, which refers to the inability of senescent cells to undergo further cell division. There is mounting evidence that cell senescence can also result in a phenotypic alteration of cells called the senescent secretory phenotype.[62,64] This phenotype is characterized by the increased production of cytokines including IL-1, IL-6, and IL-8, MMPs, and growth factors such as epidermal growth factor. The accumulation of cells expressing the senescent secretory phenotype can contribute to tissue aging and given the increased production of cytokines and MMPs in OA cartilage, may directly link aging to the development of OA (**Table 1**). There is evidence for increased MMP-3 and MMP-13 in cartilage with aging[65] as well as an age-related accumulation of collagen neoepitopes representing denatured or cleaved collagen.[66,67] Cleavage of type II collagen by MMPs has been noted in cartilage from hip joints of older individuals[66] as well as in "normal-appearing" knee cartilage taken at autopsy.[65] However, because these joints are commonly affected by OA, it is not clear if the collagen damage represents aging changes, early OA, or a continuum from aging to OA.

Cell senescence in cartilage has been associated with a decline in the ability of chondrocytes to respond to growth factors, and this could be an important contributing factor to the change in the balance of anabolic and catabolic activity seen in OA. Key matrix stimulating growth factors in cartilage include insulin-like growth factor (IGF)-I, osteogenic protein (OP)-1 (bone morphogenetic protein [BMP]-7), and TGF-β. There is substantial evidence for a decline in the chondrocyte response to IGF-I with aging[68–70] and in chondrocytes isolated from OA cartilage.[69,71] There is evidence that

Table 1
Aging changes in joint tissues and the contribution of aging to the development of OA

Aging Change	Contribution to OA
Accumulation of cells exhibiting the senescent secretory phenotype	Increased cytokine and MMP production stimulates matrix degradation
Oxidative stress/damage	Increased susceptibility to cell death and reduced matrix synthesis
Decreased levels of growth factors and decreased growth factor responsiveness	Reduced matrix synthesis and repair
Increased AGE formation	Brittle tissue with increased fatigue failure
Reduced aggrecan size and cartilage hydration and increased collagen cleavage	Reduced resiliency and tensile strength
Increased matrix calcification	Altered mechanical properties and potential activation of inflammatory signaling

Abbreviations: AGE, advanced glycation end-products; MMP, matrix metalloproteinases.
Reproduced from Anderson AS, Loeser RF. Why is osteoarthritis an age-related disease? Best Pract Res Clin Rheumatol 2010;24:15–26; with permission.

the decline in IGF-I response (or IGF-I resistance) is due to altered cell signaling. A reduced ability of IGF-I to activate cell signaling was noted in aging rat cartilage[70] and in aged equine chondrocytes.[72,73] Because IGF-I is an important autocrine survival factor in cartilage[74] the age-related decline in IGF-I signaling may play a role in age-related cell death. The expression and amount of OP-1 present in cartilage declines with age,[75] which may be related to increased DNA methylation at the OP-1 promoter.[76] Likewise, levels of TGF-β2 and TGF-β3 (but not TGF-β1) decline with age as does the level of the TGF-β receptors I and II.[77] Similar to IGF-I, age-related alterations in the TGF-β signaling pathway have been described, and these may also contribute to the development of OA.[78]

Aging in the Cartilage Matrix

Age-related changes that occur in the cartilage matrix can also contribute to the development of OA. There is evidence from knee MRI studies that cartilage thins with aging, particularly at the femoral side of the joint[79] and at the patella,[80] suggesting a gradual loss of cartilage matrix with aging. This loss could be due to a loss of cells and the reduced growth factor activity discussed above, but could also be due to something as simple as reduced water content. Articular cartilage is about 70% to 80% water. The water content in cartilage is controlled to a large extent by the presence of aggrecan, a large "aggregating" proteoglycan found in the cartilage matrix. Aggrecan contains highly sulfated glycosaminoglycan chains that are negatively charged and therefore very hydrophilic, and are responsible for the resiliency in cartilage. Age-related changes in the size, structure, and sulfation of aggrecan have been reported,[81–84] which reduce cartilage resiliency and hydration.[85]

Perhaps the best studied aging-related matrix protein modification in cartilage is the accumulation of advanced glycation end-products (AGEs). AGEs are produced by the spontaneous nonenzymatic glycation of proteins that occurs when reducing sugars including glucose, fructose, or ribose react with lysine or arginine residues.[86] Because the articular cartilage has a relatively low turnover rate, it is particularly susceptible to AGE formation that in other tissues occurs most commonly in diabetics with chronically elevated glucose levels. Type II collagen, the most abundant matrix protein in cartilage, has a half-life that has been calculated to be longer than 100 years.[87]

The accumulation of AGEs in knee cartilage has been suggested to play a role in the development of OA.[86,88] Modification of collagen by AGE formation results in increased cross-linking of collagen molecules. The most common AGE-related cross link is pentosidine, which has been found to be present in cartilage in increasing amounts with age.[87,89,90] Formation of excessive collagen cross-links affects the biomechanical properties of cartilage leading to increased stiffness, making the cartilage more brittle[91] and increasing the susceptibility of the tissue to fatigue failure.[89] Increased levels of AGEs in cartilage have also been associated with a decline in anabolic activity.[92] Although reported in a small study that used tissue removed at the time of joint replacement, amyloid has been detected in meniscal tissue from older adults,[93] suggesting additional age-related matrix changes may play a role in the development of OA.

The Role of Age-Related Oxidative Stress and Oxidative Damage in OA

The theory that aging changes in tissues are the result of oxidative damage from the chronic production of endogenous reactive oxygen species (ROS) or "free radicals" was proposed in the 1950s[94] and is still relevant to aging in joint tissues such as the articular cartilage. Human articular chondrocytes actively produce several different forms of ROS including superoxide, hydroxyl radical, hydrogen peroxide, as well as reactive nitrogen species, most notably nitric oxide.[95–97] Increased levels of intracellular ROS were recently detected in cartilage from old rats when compared with young adult rats.[98] Normally the levels of ROS are controlled by the balance of ROS production and the presence of various antioxidants. Glutathione is an important intracellular antioxidant, and when levels of ROS are in excess the ratio of oxidized to reduced glutathione is changed. Previous studies have detected an increase in oxidized glutathione with age in chondrocytes isolated from normal ankle tissue.[99] There is also evidence that levels of antioxidant enzymes, including catalase and superoxide dismutase, are present at lower levels with aging[98,100] and in OA cartilage.[101]

Because of the slow turnover of cells and matrix in cartilage, it is likely that damage from excessive ROS would accumulate over time. Evidence for oxidative damage in articular cartilage was provided by a study showing increased nitrotyrosine (a measure of oxidative damage to proteins) with aging, as well as with OA.[102] Increased levels of ROS can result in DNA damage, which has been noted in OA cartilage[103] including in mitochondrial DNA.[104] This damage can affect cell viability and matrix production. Oxidative stress can also contribute to the senescent phenotype of chondrocytes.[105] The resistance to IGF-I noted in aging and OA chondrocytes may also be related to excessive levels of ROS that have been shown to interfere with normal IGF-I signaling, resulting in reduced matrix production.[106] This situation could also occur indirectly by the production of oxidized low-density lipoproteins in cartilage, which can in turn contribute to chondrocyte senescence and reduced chondrocyte signaling.[107]

An aging-related increase in ROS levels could play an important role in the development of OA.[108] The various inflammatory mediators found to be increased in OA, including IL-1, IL-6, IL-8, TNF-α, and other cytokines, can all stimulate the further production of ROS, and ROS in turn can be involved in the increased production of MMPs.[109] In support of a role for ROS in the development of OA, the use of several antioxidant vitamins along with selenium (a glutathione peroxidase cofactor) was shown to reduce the development of OA in a mouse model,[110] N-Acetylcysteine (NAC) reduced cartilage destruction and chondrocyte apoptosis in a rat OA model[111] and in impact-loaded osteochondral explants,[112] and low intake of antioxidant vitamins has been associated with OA progression in humans.[113] However, we still have much to learn about ROS and oxidative stress in aging and OA in order to define more specific targets. In human clinical trials of chronic age-related diseases, the use of general antioxidants or antioxidant vitamins has had modest or no benefit. Defining the specific mechanisms by which ROS act, including their role in the regulation of cell signaling, should provide novel and more specific targets for therapies that would represent an advance over nondirected treatment with general antioxidants.

SUMMARY

Age is a primary risk factor for the development of OA, likely due to aging changes in cells and tissues that make the joint more susceptible to damage and less able to maintain homeostasis. OA is characterized by an imbalance between catabolic and anabolic activity driven by local production of inflammatory mediators in the cartilage and surrounding joint tissues. The senescent secretory phenotype likely contributes to this imbalance through the increased production of cytokines and MMPs and a reduced response to growth factors. More information is needed to better understand how aging changes in the bone, meniscus, and ligaments contribute to the development of OA. Oxidative stress appears to play an important role in the link between aging and OA. Understanding the basic mechanisms by which excessive ROS affect cell function at the molecular level may provide the knowledge needed to develop novel preventative treatments for OA.

REFERENCES

1. Lawrence RC, Felson DT, Helmick CG, et al. Estimates of the prevalence of arthritis and other rheumatic conditions in the United States: Part II. Arthritis Rheum 2008;58(1):26–35.
2. Murphy L, Schwartz TA, Helmick CG, et al. Lifetime risk of symptomatic knee osteoarthritis. Arthritis Rheum 2008;59(9):1207–13.
3. Lawrence JS, Bremner JM, Bier F. Osteo-arthrosis. Prevalence in the population and relationship between symptoms and x-ray changes. Ann Rheum Dis 1966; 25(1):1–24.
4. Miller ME, Rejeski WJ, Messier SP, et al. Modifiers of change in physical functioning in older adults with knee pain: the Observational Arthritis Study in Seniors (OASIS). Arthritis Rheum 2001;45(4):331–9.
5. van Saase JL, van Romunde LK, Cats A, et al. Epidemiology of osteoarthritis: Zoetermeer survey. Comparison of radiological osteoarthritis in a Dutch population with that in 10 other populations. Ann Rheum Dis 1989;48(4):271–80.
6. Zhang Y, Niu J, Kelly-Hayes M, et al. Prevalence of symptomatic hand osteoarthritis and its impact on functional status among the elderly: the Framingham Study. Am J Epidemiol 2002;156(11):1021–7.
7. Felson DT, Naimark A, Anderson J, et al. The prevalence of knee osteoarthritis in the elderly. The Framingham Osteoarthritis Study. Arthritis Rheum 1987;30(8): 914–8.
8. Jordan JM, Helmick CG, Renner JB, et al. Prevalence of knee symptoms and radiographic and symptomatic knee osteoarthritis in African Americans and Caucasians: the Johnston County Osteoarthritis Project. J Rheumatol 2007; 34(1):172–80.
9. Jordan JM, Helmick CG, Renner JB, et al. Prevalence of hip symptoms and radiographic and symptomatic hip osteoarthritis in African Americans and Caucasians: the Johnston County Osteoarthritis Project. J Rheumatol 2009; 36(4):809–15.

10. Sowers M, Lachance L, Hochberg M, et al. Radiographically defined osteoarthritis of the hand and knee in young and middle-aged African American and Caucasian women. Osteoarthritis Cartilage 2000;8(2):69–77.
11. Goldring MB, Goldring SR. Osteoarthritis. J Cell Physiol 2007;213(3):626–34.
12. Aigner T, Zhu Y, Chansky HH, et al. Reexpression of type IIA procollagen by adult articular chondrocytes in osteoarthritic cartilage. Arthritis Rheum 1999; 42(7):1443–50.
13. Sandell LJ, Aigner T. Articular cartilage and changes in arthritis. An introduction: cell biology of osteoarthritis. Arthritis Res 2001;3(2):107–13.
14. Fukui N, Ikeda Y, Ohnuki T, et al. Regional differences in chondrocyte metabolism in osteoarthritis: a detailed analysis by laser capture microdissection. Arthritis Rheum 2008;58(1):154–63.
15. Visco DM, Johnstone B, Hill MA, et al. Immunohistochemical analysis of 3-B-(−) and 7-D-4 epitope expression in canine osteoarthritis. Arthritis Rheum 1993; 36(12):1718–25.
16. Aigner T, Kim HA, Roach HI. Apoptosis in osteoarthritis. Rheum Dis Clin North Am 2004;30(3):639–53, xi.
17. Kuhn K, D'Lima DD, Hashimoto S, et al. Cell death in cartilage. Osteoarthritis Cartilage 2004;12(1):1–16.
18. Burr DB, Radin EL. Microfractures and microcracks in subchondral bone: are they relevant to osteoarthrosis? Rheum Dis Clin North Am 2003;29(4): 675–85.
19. Burr DB. The importance of subchondral bone in the progression of osteoarthritis. J Rheumatol Suppl 2004;70:77–80.
20. Mansell JP, Bailey AJ. Abnormal cancellous bone collagen metabolism in osteoarthritis. J Clin Invest 1998;101(8):1596–603.
21. Sanchez C, Deberg MA, Bellahcene A, et al. Phenotypic characterization of osteoblasts from the sclerotic zones of osteoarthritic subchondral bone. Arthritis Rheum 2008;58(2):442–55.
22. Felson DT, Chaisson CE, Hill CL, et al. The association of bone marrow lesions with pain in knee osteoarthritis. Ann Intern Med 2001;134(7):541–9.
23. Felson DT, McLaughlin S, Goggins J, et al. Bone marrow edema and its relation to progression of knee osteoarthritis. Ann Intern Med 2003;139(5 Pt 1):330–6.
24. Haywood L, McWilliams DF, Pearson CI, et al. Inflammation and angiogenesis in osteoarthritis. Arthritis Rheum 2003;48(8):2173–7.
25. Ayral X, Pickering EH, Woodworth TG, et al. Synovitis: a potential predictive factor of structural progression of medial tibiofemoral knee osteoarthritis—results of a 1 year longitudinal arthroscopic study in 422 patients. Osteoarthritis Cartilage 2005;13(5):361–7.
26. van Beuningen HM, van der Kraan PM, Arntz OJ, et al. Transforming growth factor-beta 1 stimulates articular chondrocyte proteoglycan synthesis and induces osteophyte formation in the murine knee joint. Lab Invest 1994;71(2): 279–90.
27. Spector TD, Hart DJ, Nandra D, et al. Low-level increases in serum C-reactive protein are present in early osteoarthritis of the knee and predict progressive disease. Arthritis Rheum 1997;40(4):723–7.
28. Livshits G, Zhai G, Hart DJ, et al. Interleukin-6 is a significant predictor of radiographic knee osteoarthritis: The Chingford Study. Arthritis Rheum 2009;60(7): 2037–45.
29. Felson DT. Risk factors for osteoarthritis: understanding joint vulnerability. Clin Orthop Relat Res 2004;427(Suppl):S16–21.

30. McAlindon TE, Felson DT, Zhang Y, et al. Relation of dietary intake and serum levels of vitamin D to progression of osteoarthritis of the knee among participants in the Framingham Study. Ann Intern Med 1996;125(5):353–9.

31. Chaganti RK, Parimi N, Cawthon P, et al. Association of 25-hydroxyvitamin D with prevalent osteoarthritis of the hip in elderly men: the osteoporotic fractures in men study. Arthritis Rheum 2010;62(2):511–4.

32. Gelber AC, Hochberg MC, Mead LA, et al. Joint injury in young adults and risk for subsequent knee and hip osteoarthritis. Ann Intern Med 2000;133(5): 321–8.

33. Roos H, Adalberth T, Dahlberg L, et al. Osteoarthritis of the knee after injury to the anterior cruciate ligament or meniscus: the influence of time and age. Osteoarthritis Cartilage 1995;3(4):261–7.

34. Pai YC, Rymer WZ, Chang RW, et al. Effect of age and osteoarthritis on knee proprioception. Arthritis Rheum 1997;40(12):2260–5.

35. Rosenthal AK. Calcium crystal deposition and osteoarthritis. Rheum Dis Clin North Am 2006;32(2):401–12, vii.

36. Englund M, Guermazi A, Gale D, et al. Incidental meniscal findings on knee MRI in middle-aged and elderly persons. N Engl J Med 2008;359(11):1108–15.

37. Englund M, Guermazi A, Roemer FW, et al. Meniscal tear in knees without surgery and the development of radiographic osteoarthritis among middle-aged and elderly persons: The Multicenter Osteoarthritis Study. Arthritis Rheum 2009;60(3):831–9.

38. Hill CL, Seo GS, Gale D, et al. Cruciate ligament integrity in osteoarthritis of the knee. Arthritis Rheum 2005;52(3):794–9.

39. Strocchi R, De Pasquale V, Facchini A, et al. Age-related changes in human Anterior Cruciate Ligament (ACL) collagen fibrils. Archivio italiano di anatomia ed embriologia. Ital J Anat Embryol 1996;101(4):213–20.

40. Felson DT, Neogi T. Osteoarthritis: is it a disease of cartilage or of bone? Arthritis Rheum 2004;50(2):341–4.

41. Lo GH, Hunter DJ, Nevitt M, et al. Strong association of MRI meniscal derangement and bone marrow lesions in knee osteoarthritis: data from the osteoarthritis initiative. Osteoarthritis Cartilage 2009;17(6):743–7.

42. Hunter DJ, Gerstenfeld L, Bishop G, et al. Bone marrow lesions from osteoarthritis knees are characterized by sclerotic bone that is less well mineralized. Arthritis Res Ther 2009;11(1):R11.

43. Baranyay FJ, Wang Y, Wluka AE, et al. Association of bone marrow lesions with knee structures and risk factors for bone marrow lesions in the knees of clinically healthy, community-based adults. Semin Arthritis Rheum 2007;37(2):112–8.

44. Felson DT, Anderson JJ, Naimark A, et al. The prevalence of chondrocalcinosis in the elderly and its association with knee osteoarthritis: the Framingham Study. J Rheumatol 1989;16(9):1241–5.

45. Doherty M, Dieppe P. Clinical aspects of calcium pyrophosphate dihydrate crystal deposition. Rheum Dis Clin North Am 1988;14(2):395–414.

46. Richette P, Bardin T, Doherty M. An update on the epidemiology of calcium pyrophosphate dihydrate crystal deposition disease. Rheumatology (Oxford) 2009; 48(7):711–5.

47. Neame RL, Carr AJ, Muir K, et al. UK community prevalence of knee chondrocalcinosis: evidence that correlation with osteoarthritis is through a shared association with osteophyte. Ann Rheum Dis 2003;62(6):513–8.

48. Nalbant S, Martinez JA, Kitumnuaypong T, et al. Synovial fluid features and their relations to osteoarthritis severity: new findings from sequential studies. Osteoarthritis Cartilage 2003;11(1):50–4.
49. Liu-Bryan R, Pritzker K, Firestein GS, et al. TLR2 signaling in chondrocytes drives calcium pyrophosphate dihydrate and monosodium urate crystal-induced nitric oxide generation. J Immunol 2005;174(8):5016–23.
50. Punzi L, Ramonda R, Sfriso P. Erosive osteoarthritis. Best Pract Res Clin Rheumatol 2004;18(5):739–58.
51. Vlychou M, Koutroumpas A, Malizos K, et al. Ultrasonographic evidence of inflammation is frequent in hands of patients with erosive osteoarthritis. Osteoarthritis Cartilage 2009;17(10):1283–7.
52. Aigner T, Hemmel M, Neureiter D, et al. Apoptotic cell death is not a widespread phenomenon in normal aging and osteoarthritis human articular knee cartilage: a study of proliferation, programmed cell death (apoptosis), and viability of chondrocytes in normal and osteoarthritic human knee cartilage. Arthritis Rheum 2001;44(6):1304–12.
53. Dowthwaite GP, Bishop JC, Redman SN, et al. The surface of articular cartilage contains a progenitor cell population. J Cell Sci 2004;117(Pt 6):889–97.
54. Alsalameh S, Amin R, Gemba T, et al. Identification of mesenchymal progenitor cells in normal and osteoarthritic human articular cartilage. Arthritis Rheum 2004;50(5):1522–32.
55. Horton WE Jr, Feng L, Adams C. Chondrocyte apoptosis in development, aging and disease. Matrix Biol 1998;17(2):107–15.
56. Vignon E, Arlot M, Patricot LM, et al. The cell density of human femoral head cartilage. Clin Orthop 1976;121(121):303–8.
57. Adams CS, Horton WE Jr. Chondrocyte apoptosis increases with age in the articular cartilage of adult animals. Anat Rec 1998;250(4):418–25.
58. Taniguchi N, Carames B, Ronfani L, et al. Aging-related loss of the chromatin protein HMGB2 in articular cartilage is linked to reduced cellularity and osteoarthritis. Proc Natl Acad Sci U S A 2009;106(4):1181–6.
59. Martin JA, Buckwalter JA. Telomere erosion and senescence in human articular cartilage chondrocytes. J Gerontol A Biol Sci Med Sci 2001;56(4):B172–9.
60. Hayflick L. Intracellular determinants of cell aging. Mech Ageing Dev 1984;28(2–3):177–85.
61. Itahana K, Campisi J, Dimri GP. Mechanisms of cellular senescence in human and mouse cells. Biogerontology 2004;5(1):1–10.
62. Campisi J. Senescent cells, tumor suppression, and organismal aging: good citizens, bad neighbors. Cell 2005;120(4):513–22.
63. Dai SM, Shan ZZ, Nakamura H, et al. Catabolic stress induces features of chondrocyte senescence through overexpression of caveolin 1: possible involvement of caveolin 1-induced down-regulation of articular chondrocytes in the pathogenesis of osteoarthritis. Arthritis Rheum 2006;54(3):818–31.
64. Campisi J, d'Adda di Fagagna F. Cellular senescence: when bad things happen to good cells. Nat Rev Mol Cell Biol 2007;8(9):729–40.
65. Wu W, Billinghurst RC, Pidoux I, et al. Sites of collagenase cleavage and denaturation of type II collagen in aging and osteoarthritic articular cartilage and their relationship to the distribution of matrix metalloproteinase 1 and matrix metalloproteinase 13. Arthritis Rheum 2002;46(8):2087–94.
66. Hollander AP, Pidoux I, Reiner A, et al. Damage to type II collagen in aging and osteoarthritis starts at the articular surface, originates around chondrocytes, and

extends into the cartilage with progressive degeneration. J Clin Invest 1995; 96(6):2859–69.

67. Aurich M, Poole AR, Reiner A, et al. Matrix homeostasis in aging normal human ankle cartilage. Arthritis Rheum 2002;46(11):2903–10.

68. Martin JA, Ellerbroek SM, Buckwalter JA. Age-related decline in chondrocyte response to insulin-like growth factor-I: the role of growth factor binding proteins. J Orthop Res 1997;15(4):491–8.

69. Loeser RF, Shanker G, Carlson CS, et al. Reduction in the chondrocyte response to insulin-like growth factor 1 in aging and osteoarthritis: studies in a non-human primate model of naturally occurring disease. Arthritis Rheum 2000;43(9): 2110–20.

70. Messai H, Duchossoy Y, Khatib A, et al. Articular chondrocytes from aging rats respond poorly to insulin-like growth factor-1: an altered signaling pathway. Mech Ageing Dev 2000;115(1–2):21–37.

71. Dore S, Pelletier JP, DiBattista JA, et al. Human osteoarthritic chondrocytes possess an increased number of insulin-like growth factor 1 binding sites but are unresponsive to its stimulation. Possible role of IGF-1-binding proteins. Arthritis Rheum 1994;37(2):253–63.

72. Fortier LA, Miller BJ. Signaling through the small G-protein Cdc42 is involved in insulin-like growth factor-I resistance in aging articular chondrocytes. J Orthop Res 2006;24(8):1765–72.

73. Boehm AK, Seth M, Mayr KG, et al. Hsp90 mediates insulin-like growth factor 1 and interleukin-1beta signaling in an age-dependent manner in equine articular chondrocytes. Arthritis Rheum 2007;56(7):2335–43.

74. Loeser RF, Shanker G. Autocrine stimulation by insulin-like growth factor 1 and insulin-like growth factor 2 mediates chondrocyte survival in vitro. Arthritis Rheum 2000;43(7):1552–9.

75. Chubinskaya S, Kumar B, Merrihew C, et al. Age-related changes in cartilage endogenous osteogenic protein-1 (OP-1). Biochim Biophys Acta 2002; 1588(2):126–34.

76. Loeser RF, Im HJ, Richardson B, et al. Methylation of the OP-1 promoter: potential role in the age-related decline in OP-1 expression in cartilage. Osteoarthritis Cartilage 2009;17(4):513–7.

77. Blaney Davidson EN, Scharstuhl A, Vitters EL, et al. Reduced transforming growth factor-beta signaling in cartilage of old mice: role in impaired repair capacity. Arthritis Res Ther 2005;7(6):R1338–47.

78. van der Kraan PM, Blaney Davidson EN, van den Berg WB. A role for age-related changes in TGFbeta signaling in aberrant chondrocyte differentiation and osteoarthritis. Arthritis Res Ther 2010;12(1):201.

79. Hudelmaier M, Glaser C, Hohe J, et al. Age-related changes in the morphology and deformational behavior of knee joint cartilage. Arthritis Rheum 2001;44(11): 2556–61.

80. Ding C, Cicuttini F, Scott F, et al. Association between age and knee structural change: a cross sectional MRI based study. Ann Rheum Dis 2005;64(4): 549–55.

81. Buckwalter JA, Roughley PJ, Rosenberg LC. Age-related changes in cartilage proteoglycans: quantitative electron microscopic studies. Microsc Res Tech 1994;28(5):398–408.

82. Dudhia J, Davidson CM, Wells TM, et al. Age-related changes in the content of the C-terminal region of aggrecan in human articular cartilage. Biochem J 1996; 313(Pt 3):933–40.

83. Bayliss MT, Osborne D, Woodhouse S, et al. Sulfation of chondroitin sulfate in human articular cartilage. The effect of age, topographical position, and zone of cartilage on tissue composition. J Biol Chem 1999;274(22): 15892–900.
84. Wells T, Davidson C, Morgelin M, et al. Age-related changes in the composition, the molecular stoichiometry and the stability of proteoglycan aggregates extracted from human articular cartilage. Biochem J 2003;370(Pt 1):69–79.
85. Grushko G, Schneiderman R, Maroudas A. Some biochemical and biophysical parameters for the study of the pathogenesis of osteoarthritis: a comparison between the processes of ageing and degeneration in human hip cartilage. Connect Tissue Res 1989;19(2–4):149–76.
86. Verzijl N, Bank RA, TeKoppele JM, et al. AGEing and osteoarthritis: a different perspective. Curr Opin Rheumatol 2003;15(5):616–22.
87. Verzijl N, DeGroot J, Thorpe SR, et al. Effect of collagen turnover on the accumulation of advanced glycation endproducts. J Biol Chem 2000;275: 39027–31.
88. DeGroot J, Verzijl N, Wenting-van Wijk MJ, et al. Accumulation of advanced glycation end products as a molecular mechanism for aging as a risk factor in osteoarthritis. Arthritis Rheum 2004;50(4):1207–15.
89. Bank RA, Bayliss MT, Lafeber FP, et al. Ageing and zonal variation in post-translational modification of collagen in normal human articular cartilage. The age-related increase in non-enzymatic glycation affects biomechanical properties of cartilage. Biochem J 1998;330(Pt 1):345–51.
90. Verzijl N, DeGroot J, Ben ZC, et al. Crosslinking by advanced glycation end products increases the stiffness of the collagen network in human articular cartilage: a possible mechanism through which age is a risk factor for osteoarthritis. Arthritis Rheum 2002;46(1):114–23.
91. Chen AC, Temple MM, Ng DM, et al. Induction of advanced glycation end products and alterations of the tensile properties of articular cartilage. Arthritis Rheum 2002;46(12):3212–7.
92. DeGroot J, Verzijl N, Bank RA, et al. Age-related decrease in proteoglycan synthesis of human articular chondrocytes: the role of nonenzymatic glycation. Arthritis Rheum 1999;42(5):1003–9.
93. Solomon A, Murphy CL, Kestler D, et al. Amyloid contained in the knee joint meniscus is formed from apolipoprotein A-I. Arthritis Rheum 2006;54(11): 3545–50.
94. Harman D. Aging: a theory based on free radical and radiation chemistry. J Gerontol 1956;11:298–300.
95. Studer R, Jaffurs D, Stefanovic-Racic M, et al. Nitric oxide in osteoarthritis. Osteoarthritis Cartilage 1999;7(4):377–9.
96. Hiran TS, Moulton PJ, Hancock JT. Detection of superoxide and NADPH oxidase in porcine articular chondrocytes. Free Radic Biol Med 1997;23(5):736–43.
97. Tiku ML, Shah R, Allison GT. Evidence linking chondrocyte lipid peroxidation to cartilage matrix protein degradation: Possible role in cartilage aging and the pathogenesis of osteoarthritis. J Biol Chem 2000;275:20069–76.
98. Jallali N, Ridha H, Thrasivoulou C, et al. Vulnerability to ROS-induced cell death in ageing articular cartilage: the role of antioxidant enzyme activity. Osteoarthritis Cartilage 2005;13(7):614–22.
99. Del Carlo M Jr, Loeser RF. Increased oxidative stress with aging reduces chondrocyte survival: correlation with intracellular glutathione levels. Arthritis Rheum 2003;48(12):3419–30.

100. Ruiz-Romero C, Calamia V, Mateos J, et al. Mitochondrial dysregulation of osteoarthritic human articular chondrocytes analyzed by proteomics: a decrease in mitochondrial superoxide dismutase points to a redox imbalance. Mol Cell Proteomics 2008;8(1):179–89.

101. Aigner T, Fundel K, Saas J, et al. Large-scale gene expression profiling reveals major pathogenetic pathways of cartilage degeneration in osteoarthritis. Arthritis Rheum 2006;54(11):3533–44.

102. Loeser RF, Carlson CS, Carlo MD, et al. Detection of nitrotyrosine in aging and osteoarthritic cartilage: correlation of oxidative damage with the presence of interleukin-1beta and with chondrocyte resistance to insulin-like growth factor 1. Arthritis Rheum 2002;46(9):2349–57.

103. Davies CM, Guilak F, Weinberg JB, et al. Reactive nitrogen and oxygen species in interleukin-1-mediated DNA damage associated with osteoarthritis. Osteoarthritis Cartilage 2008;16(5):624–30.

104. Grishko VI, Ho R, Wilson GL, et al. Diminished mitochondrial DNA integrity and repair capacity in OA chondrocytes. Osteoarthritis Cartilage 2009;17(1):107–13.

105. Yudoh K, Nguyen T, Nakamura H, et al. Potential involvement of oxidative stress in cartilage senescence and development of osteoarthritis: oxidative stress induces chondrocyte telomere instability and downregulation of chondrocyte function. Arthritis Res Ther 2005;7(2):R380–91.

106. Yin W, Park JI, Loeser RF. Oxidative stress inhibits insulin-like growth factor-I induction of chondrocyte proteoglycan synthesis through differential regulation of phosphatidylinositol 3-Kinase-Akt and MEK-ERK MAPK signaling pathways. J Biol Chem 2009;284(46):31972–81.

107. Zushi S, Akagi M, Kishimoto H, et al. Induction of bovine articular chondrocyte senescence with oxidized low-density lipoprotein through lectin-like oxidized low-density lipoprotein receptor 1. Arthritis Rheum 2009;60(10):3007–16.

108. Henrotin YE, Bruckner P, Pujol JP. The role of reactive oxygen species in homeostasis and degradation of cartilage. Osteoarthritis Cartilage 2003;11(10): 747–55.

109. Nelson KK, Melendez JA. Mitochondrial redox control of matrix metalloproteinases. Free Radic Biol Med 2004;37(6):768–84.

110. Kurz B, Jost B, Schunke M. Dietary vitamins and selenium diminish the development of mechanically induced osteoarthritis and increase the expression of antioxidative enzymes in the knee joint of STR/1N mice. Osteoarthritis Cartilage 2002;10(2):119–26.

111. Nakagawa S, Arai Y, Mazda O, et al. N-acetylcysteine prevents nitric oxide-induced chondrocyte apoptosis and cartilage degeneration in an experimental model of osteoarthritis. J Orthop Res 2010;28(2):156–63.

112. Martin JA, McCabe D, Walter M, et al. N-acetylcysteine inhibits post-impact chondrocyte death in osteochondral explants. J Bone Joint Surg Am 2009; 91(8):1890–7.

113. McAlindon TE, Jacques P, Zhang Y, et al. Do antioxidant micronutrients protect against the development and progression of knee osteoarthritis? Arthritis Rheum 1996;39(4):648–56.

The Contribution of Osteoarthritis to Functional Limitations and Disability

Christine M. McDonough, PhD, PT[a,b,*], Alan M. Jette, PhD, PT[a]

KEYWORDS

- Osteoarthritis • Arthritis • Function • Disability • Activity
- Participation • Disablement

It is widely stated that arthritis is the leading cause of disability among adults.[1–9] Indeed, there is no question that osteoarthritis (OA) in particular is related to disability as adults age. The risk of OA increases with age, so that by the age of 80 years radiographic evidence of joint degeneration is found in nearly everyone.[10] However, there is much that remains unknown about the specific contributions of osteoarthritis and intervening variables to the development of disability. Ferrucci and colleagues[11] revealed that as people age, a larger proportion of disability occurs along a slower, progressive course compared with more rapid onset, "catastrophic disability." Research supports the characterization of OA as one example of a condition that is characterized by the slow progression of disability.[12–15]

OA pathology results in the degeneration of cartilage, bone, and soft tissues integral to joints; most commonly the hand, knee, hip, spine, and foot. Discordance between OA pathology and resultant disability highlight opportunities to identify modifiable factors in the pathway from pathology to disability. Although OA is associated with

Dr McDonough is supported by a New Investigator Fellowship Training Initiative in Health Services Research award from the Foundation for Physical Therapy. This work was supported, in part, by the Boston Claude D. Pepper Older Americans Independence Center (P30-AG031679).

Commercial support/conflicts statement: None.

[a] Department of Health Policy and Management, Health & Disability Research Institute, Boston University School of Public Health, 715 Albany Street, T5W, Boston, MA 02118, USA

[b] The Dartmouth Institute for Health Policy and Clinical Practice, Dartmouth College, 30 Lafayette Street, 1st Floor Lebanon, NH 03766, USA

* Corresponding author. Department of Health Policy and Management, Health & Disability Research Institute, Boston University School of Public Health, 715 Albany Street, T5W, Boston, MA 02118.

E-mail address: cmm@bu.edu

Clin Geriatr Med 26 (2010) 387–399
doi:10.1016/j.cger.2010.04.001
0749-0690/10/$ – see front matter © 2010 Elsevier Inc. All rights reserved.

joint-related symptoms such as pain and stiffness, there is wide variation in symptoms for those with radiographic evidence of joint degeneration changes, and many with radiographic changes report no pain.[16]

Studies of OA and disability use a range of definitions for OA and for disability, and this presents challenges to summarizing and interpreting the literature. Often, diagnosis of OA is made based on radiographic signs and joint symptoms; however, the former is considered to be associated with later stages of disease. In previous work, investigators have highlighted the importance of a disablement conceptual framework to guide the investigation of disability and its determinants.[17] Therefore, to guide this analysis of the importance of OA in the development of disability, the Disablement Model developed by Verbrugge and Jette, based on the seminal work by Nagi, is used in this article.[18–20] The Disablement Model (**Fig. 1**) presents the main pathway for the development of disability with factors affecting progression including risk factors, extra-individual factors, and intra-individual factors. Because the pathway represents a continuum from cellular to societal level effects, the threshold for transition from one element to another is debatable. The pathway is reviewed in the next section, and elements of OA are related to the levels of the pathway to facilitate the review and discussion.

THE MAIN PATHWAY

The main disablement pathway progresses from pathology to impairments, to functional limitations, and finally to disability.

"*Pathology* refers to biochemical or physiologic abnormalities that are detected and labeled as disease, injury, or congenital/developmental conditions."[20] OA pathology includes biologic and physiologic changes to the hyaline cartilage and neighboring bone, synovial fluid and soft tissue, ligaments and muscle. The development of sclerotic changes in subchondral bone tissue, osteophyte growth, and synovial tissue proliferation are examples of pathology in OA.

"*Impairments* are dysfunctions and significant structural abnormalities" that occur at the level of the body systems or organs, and are "the functional consequence of pathology."[20] Abnormalities related to OA that reach the level of impairment may include joint swelling, deformity or malalignment, decreased strength, limitations in range of motion, abnormalities of gait, and symptoms such as pain and stiffness.

Functional limitations occur at the level of the person and represent limitations in executing specific mental or physical actions or tasks. Examples of functional limitations include restrictions in walking, picking up items from the floor, and climbing stairs.

Disability is defined as limitations, difficulty, or inability to do more complex behaviors or activities that are performed within a social, cultural, or physical context. Disability behaviors reflect what a person does in daily life and range from activities of daily living (ADL) such as dressing, doing household chores and errands, to fulfilling social roles in such contexts of work, community, and family.

The Disablement Model includes outcomes beyond disability such as hospitalization, inability to live alone, and death, and pathways from disability to functional limitations, impairments, and pathology. These are important considerations for researchers undertaking to investigate the causal mechanisms involved in the process.

THE FACTORS

To facilitate understanding and investigation of the causal mechanisms in the progression from one stage of disablement to another, the Disablement Model identifies

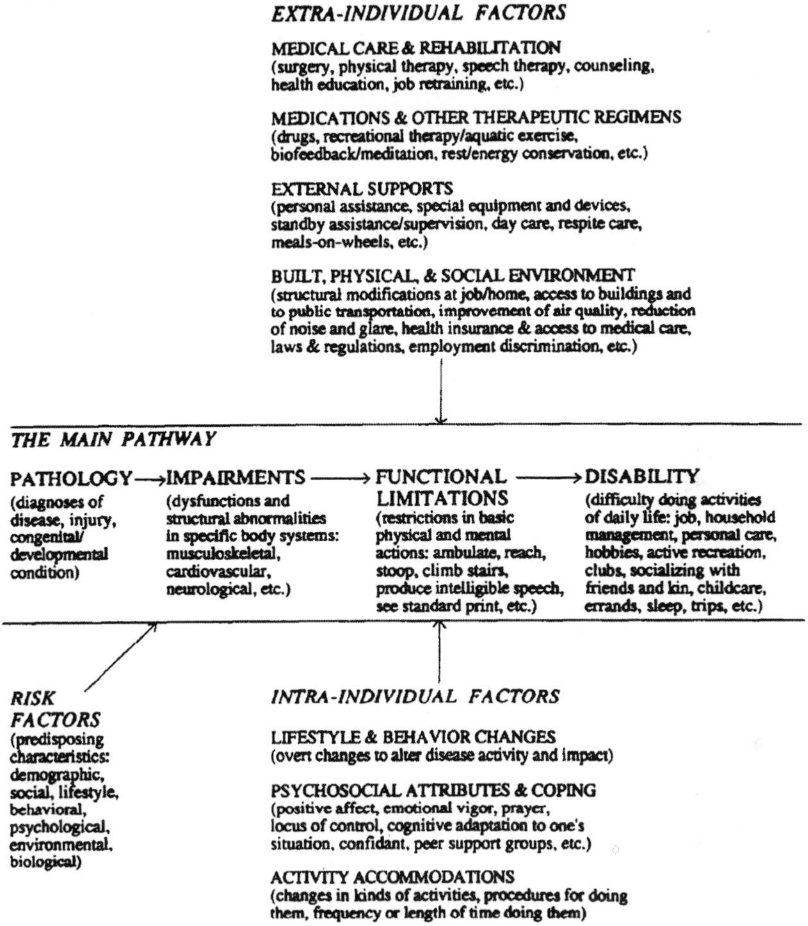

EXTRA-INDIVIDUAL FACTORS

MEDICAL CARE & REHABILITATION
(surgery, physical therapy, speech therapy, counseling,
health education, job retraining, etc.)

MEDICATIONS & OTHER THERAPEUTIC REGIMENS
(drugs, recreational therapy/aquatic exercise,
biofeedback/meditation, rest/energy conservation, etc.)

EXTERNAL SUPPORTS
(personal assistance, special equipment and devices,
standby assistance/supervision, day care, respite care,
meals-on-wheels, etc.)

BUILT, PHYSICAL, & SOCIAL ENVIRONMENT
(structural modifications at job/home, access to buildings and
to public transportation, improvement of air quality, reduction
of noise and glare, health insurance & access to medical care,
laws & regulations, employment discrimination, etc.)

THE MAIN PATHWAY

PATHOLOGY→	IMPAIRMENTS ——→	FUNCTIONAL ——→ LIMITATIONS	DISABILITY
(diagnoses of disease, injury, congenital/ developmental condition)	(dysfunctions and structural abnormalities in specific body systems: musculoskeletal, cardiovascular, neurological, etc.)	(restrictions in basic physical and mental actions: ambulate, reach, stoop, climb stairs, produce intelligible speech, see standard print, etc.)	(difficulty doing activities of daily life: job, household management, personal care, hobbies, active recreation, friends and kin, childcare, errands, sleep, trips, etc.)

RISK FACTORS
(predisposing characteristics: demographic, social, lifestyle, behavioral, psychological, environmental, biological)

INTRA-INDIVIDUAL FACTORS

LIFESTYLE & BEHAVIOR CHANGES
(overt changes to alter disease activity and impact)

PSYCHOSOCIAL ATTRIBUTES & COPING
(positive affect, emotional vigor, prayer,
locus of control, cognitive adaptation to one's
situation, confidant, peer support groups, etc.)

ACTIVITY ACCOMMODATIONS
(changes in kinds of activities, procedures for doing
them, frequency or length of time doing them)

Fig. 1. Verbrugge and Jette's disablement model. (*From* Verbrugge LM, Jette AM. The disablement process. Soc Sci Med 1994;38:4; with permission.)

several categories of intervening factors: predisposing risk factors, intra-individual intervening factors, and extra-individual intervening factors.

Predisposing risk factors are preexisting characteristics of the individual that can affect the presence of impairment, functional limitation, and disability, and its severity. These characteristics range from sociodemographic, lifestyle, psychological, and biologic factors and exist before the onset of the disablement process.

Intra-individual intervening factors aim to affect the disease and its repercussions on degree of impairment, functional limitation, and disability, and include the following categories: lifestyle and behavior changes; psychosocial attributes and coping mechanisms; and individual accommodations to activity (changing the length of time spent doing an activity or the types of activities done).

Extra-individual intervening factors include "medical care and rehabilitation, medications & other therapeutic regimens, external supports, and built, physical, and social environment" factors.[20] The terms buffers and exacerbators are used to describe the potential positive or negative effects of the existing environment or active interventions.

In arthritis research, disability outcomes may include variables ranging from the level of impairment (symptoms, weakness, and malalignment) to that of disability (difficulty doing activities at the intersection of person and environment). Similarly, OA may be defined as joint pain, or joint pain associated with radiographic changes. It should be noted that arthritis as defined in large national studies often includes other conditions such as rheumatoid arthritis, spinal disorders, and arthropathies. This presents challenges for interpreting the literature as it relates to osteoarthritis. However, for most persons in the larger arthritis category, the form of arthritis that they experience is osteoarthritis. An example of the prevalence estimates from 1 national study is provided. Verbrugge and colleagues[21] estimated that 43.7% of the US population has arthritis, and further stratified prevalence rates as: 34.8% of men older than 55 years have arthritis, and 32.7% have osteoarthritis. Similarly the prevalence rates for women older than 55 years were 50.6% for arthritis and 47.1% for osteoarthritis. Therefore, the authors have included relevant studies using the broader definition of arthritis in this review when it was found that they provided important information about the relationship between arthritis and functional limitations and disability that may guide future work specific to osteoarthritis. The authors use the term osteoarthritis or OA to represent the more specific diagnosis when appropriate, and use the term arthritis to denote the larger category that includes conditions other than osteoarthritis. The authors focus on the 2 elements to the right in the main pathway because together they represent what is meant by many when they refer to "disability." In doing so, the risk factors, intra-individual factors, and extra-individual factors that affect the relationship between these elements are addressed. Gaps in knowledge are highlighted and directions for future inquiry are proposed.

THE CONTRIBUTION OF ARTHRITIS TO FUNCTIONAL LIMITATIONS AND DISABILITY

Many cross-sectional studies have demonstrated a substantial relationship between arthritis and functional limitations and disability, a selection of which are highlighted here. Fewer studies address the contribution of osteoarthritis to disability.

Research indicates that the effect of arthritis on disability is greater on physical functional limitations than on more complex social and role activities.[22] Verbrugge and colleagues[21] compared levels of functional limitation and disability for those with and without arthritis in a nationally representative sample living in the United States using data from the Supplement on Aging of the 1984 National Health Interview Survey. This study investigated the relationship between more than 20 indicators of functional limitation and disability including walking, motions and strength (eg, reaching, lifting, standing), personal care, and household activities among those with a range of arthritic conditions. Across all of these measures, members of this sample with arthritis experienced more disability than those who did not, and the effect of arthritis was greater on functional limitations than on disability, represented by more complex social role activities. Comparing the effect of various health conditions, results from the Women's Health and Aging Study have also revealed that women reporting "a physician with a diagnosis of arthritis" were significantly more likely to report difficulty in 13 of 15 functional tasks and activities.[23]

Employing the World Health Organization's Disability Assessment Schedule, and the National Comorbidity Survey Replication, Merikangas and colleagues[24] used regression analysis to estimate the effect of specific conditions on disability days. Arthritis more generally accounted for the third largest number of disability days

(374.6 million days per year), after back/neck pain (1167.8 million days per year) and major depressive disorder (386.6 million days per year).

Verbrugge and colleagues[25] provided detail on the emerging picture of the contribution of arthritis to functional limitations and disability by analyzing the 1994–95 National Health Interview's Disability Supplement Phase I. In this "profile of arthritis disability," those with arthritis (including osteo, rheumatoid, spinal, and other arthropathies), had a slower progression of milder disabilities than persons with disabilities from other conditions. This "profile of arthritis disability" is consistent with Ferrucci and colleagues' concept of "progressive disability" characterized by a slower more progressive course compared with more rapid onset seen in "catastrophic disability."

A second profile of arthritis disability used the National Health Interview's Disability Supplement Phase II to compare a range of functional limitations and disability for persons who attributed their disability to arthritis (including osteo, rheumatoid, spinal, and other arthropathies) against those with disability attributed to other conditions.[9] They reported that those with arthritis were more likely to be older, female, and less likely to be working than those with other disabling conditions, and to report that they were unable to work because of their health. Overall, arthritis-disabled persons experienced more disability across a wider range of activities than other-disabled persons. With regard to participation in social activities, arthritis-disabled persons reported traveling long distances less often, using a vehicle for transportation less often, going out fewer days per week, and were less likely to report working at a job. This study provided new knowledge about the functional course for those with arthritis in middle age, and revealed that they experienced functional limitations and disability earlier than those without arthritis.

In longitudinal research, Song and colleagues[8] estimated the population effect of arthritis using data from the nationally representative National Health and Retirement Survey. Arthritis was identified when respondents answered yes to the question, "Have you ever had or has a doctor ever told you that you have arthritis or rheumatism?" Investigators used multiple logistic regression analysis to compare the incidence of new functional limitation or disability (preparing meals, grocery shopping, managing money, taking medications, using the telephone). Consistent with previous studies, investigators noted that risk factors for incident disability among persons 65 years and older were demographic factors, age, comorbid conditions, physical limitations, health behaviors (tobacco and alcohol use, and physical activity), and socioeconomic factors, and they adjusted for them in the analysis. Song and colleagues[8] conclude from their findings, "Almost 1 in every 4 new cases of ADL disability was due to arthritis (adjusted population attributable fraction 23.7%)." In his editorial comment, Covinsky wrote, "Although Song and colleagues demonstrated that in a statistical sense almost 25% of disability is attributable to arthritis, it would not be correct to claim that arthritis is the cause of disability in 1 of 4 individuals with ADL dependence. In contrast, a conclusion stating that arthritis is the contributing cause in 75% of patients with ADL disability, and on average accounts for one-third of the disability is clinically very plausible."[1]

A recent longitudinal study with 10-year follow-up from the Health and Retirement Study addressed the need to investigate the role of arthritis (as defined by the response to the same general arthritis question used in Song and colleagues' study) earlier in life in the later development of functional limitations (walking and climbing stairs) or disability (bathing, dressing, transfers, eating, and toileting).[2] The baseline results indicated that those with arthritis were significantly more likely to be older, female, of lower socioeconomic status, and have comorbid conditions (eg, hypertension, depressive symptoms, cancer, or diabetes). After adjusting for age, sex, socioeconomic status, comorbid conditions, body mass index, smoking, depression, physical activity, difficulty jogging 1 mile, and difficulty climbing stairs, investigators found that those with arthritis had significantly higher risk of developing functional limitations (30% vs 16%) or difficulty with ADL function (13% vs 5%) over 10 years. The adjusted odds ratio for mobility or ADL difficulty for those with arthritis compared with those without arthritis was 1.63 (1.43–1.86). Investigators also calculated odds ratios for those with arthritis only and those without arthritis and at least 1 other condition compared with those with no arthritis or other conditions. The adjusted odds ratios for those with arthritis and those with at least 1 other condition were 1.91 (1.59–2.44) and 1.74 (1.46–2.08), respectively. This study provided new knowledge about the course of functional limitations and disability over a long period in those who experience arthritis in middle age.

THE CONTRIBUTION OF OSTEOARTHRITIS TO FUNCTIONAL LIMITATIONS AND DISABILITY

Guccione and colleagues[26] used logistic regression to estimate the odds of dependence in 7 functional tasks and activities. They found that knee OA was among the most disabling conditions, and was associated with the most limitation in walking and climbing stairs. The adjusted percentage of disability attributable to OA was approximately 16%, and equal to or higher than 9 other major conditions in 4 out of the 7 functional items (walking, carrying, climbing stairs, and housekeeping).

One approach to estimating the overall burden of conditions on disability used by the World Health Organization is the Disability Adjusted Life Year (DALY). DALYs take into account the length of life and time spent with disability, by estimating the duration of healthy life lost as a result of a condition. Using data from 1990, and projecting the effect of OA in 2000, Reginster and colleagues[27] reported that OA had the fourth greatest impact on disability, following ischemic heart disease, cerebrovascular disease, and all musculoskeletal disease.

Using data from a nationwide survey in France, Fautrel and colleagues[28] used reported limitation rates to calculate standardized limitation rate ratios (SLRRs) for those with OA compared with age- and sex-matched controls. They found that persons with OA reported limitations in mobility 4.5 to 6 times more frequently than those without. Among those with OA, 61% reported limitation in mobility outside the home compared with 10.2% reported by controls. Inside the home, 12.8% of those with OA reported mobility limitations compared with 2.8% of controls. Similar patterns with smaller differences were observed for ADL such as shopping and housecleaning. SLRRs ranged from 1.6 for dressing and sports to 6.0 for mobility outside the home.

Zhang and colleagues[29] found persons with hand OA experienced significant functional limitations in functions involving the hands compared with those who did not have hand OA, including writing, gripping, and manipulating small objects.

In summary, a range of approaches has been used to characterize the unequivocal contribution of the presence of arthritis generally and OA in particular, to the development of functional limitations and disability. Evidence overwhelmingly supports a significant, moderate independent contribution of arthritis to the onset and progression of functional limitations and disability. The authors now consider a range of important risk and intervening factors that have been shown to mediate the effect of arthritis to a greater or lesser degree on loss of function and the development of disability.

FACTORS INFLUENCING THE COURSE OF DISABLEMENT
Overview of Factors

In their paper summarizing a 1999 NIH Scientific Conference, Felson and colleagues[5] highlighted the differences in risk factors for OA pathology and the development of functional limitations and disability succinctly: "Whereas osteoarthritis is associated with increasing age, obesity, injury, previous deformity, and ligamentous laxity, the broader clinical problem, of musculoskeletal pain and disability is predicted by increasing age; osteoarthritis; obesity; lack of exercise; low personal self-efficacy; comorbid conditions caused by smoking, alcohol, and other risk factors; depression; low educational level; and poor socioeconomic status." Indeed, a more recent review identifies structural manifestations of pathology and symptoms (eg, knee joint laxity, decreased muscle strength, decreased range of motion); visual and cognitive deficits; comorbidity; overweight; psychological and social factors including anxiety, depression, fatigue, poor self-efficacy, and social support; health behaviors and sociodemographic factors as predictive factors.[30] This report is consistent with previous work except that van Dijk and colleagues[15] note that increased level of aerobic exercise is a protective factor. The authors review selected individual studies that support these findings, and focus more on modifiable factors.

Predisposing and Intra-individual Risk Factors

Dunlop and colleagues[31] used longitudinal data from a national probability sample and multiple logistic regression to investigate risk factors for functional decline. Functional decline was associated with female gender and race for those with arthritis. Additional risk factors included age, cognitive and visual impairment, symptoms of depression, stroke, and physical limitations. The chief finding was that lack of regular vigorous exercise could predict an important increased risk of decline.[31]

Impairment-level factors

In cross-sectional analysis of data from a community sample, Wilkie and colleagues[32] used logistic regression to investigate the association between a range of risk factors and disability. Their findings indicated that self-reported joint-level impairment was associated with functional limitations and disability, and that a stronger association existed between functional limitations and disability than between impairment and disability. Other cross-sectional analyses support the relationship between knee pain and functional limitations.[33–35]

Sharma and colleagues[14] used multiple measures of physical function and logistic regression to investigate factors predictive of functional decline over 3 years in this study of community-dwelling adults with knee osteoarthritis. They found that baseline knee laxity, knee pain intensity, and baseline to 18-month increase in knee pain increased risk of functional decline as measured by the Western Ontario McMaster University Osteoarthritis Index. Impaired position sense was associated with decline in the ability to perform sit-to-stand from a chair. In other studies, baseline pain and increase in pain predicted functional limitations.[12,36] In their recent longitudinal study of adults with hip and knee OA, van Dijk and colleagues found little overall change in physical function, but important variation at the individual level. Factors predictive of decline included decrements of strength and range of motion, and increased pain.

Ling and colleagues[7] found that knee extensor strength was predictive of transition to new functional limitations in a longitudinal cohort of women using data from the Women's Health and Aging Study. Miller and colleagues[37] used mixed effects repeated measures analysis of covariance to investigate the relationship between baseline radiographic evidence of OA, knee strength, and knee pain, and functional outcomes (ambulation test, transfer test, and self-report of physical function). They reported that although baseline radiographic evidence of OA was associated with decline in all measures of physical function initially, this relationship was not significant when baseline levels of knee pain and knee strength were included in the model. This study could not address the temporal pattern of these 3 impairment-level factors. Jinks and colleagues[38] found that despite resolved knee pain at 3-year follow-up, physical function had made minimal improvement.

Research into the relationship between joint pain, depression, and physical function illustrates the opportunities for improved understanding of the relative contribution to functional limitations and disability and timing of its effects. Machado and colleagues[39] reported that the relationship between baseline pain and downstream disability was mediated by depressive symptoms. They demonstrated that physical symptoms affect higher level disability through lower level physical functional limitations and depressive symptoms.

In summary, with respect to important risk factors for the development of functional limitations and disability among those with OA, the evidence provides strong support for the role of physical impairments in the development of functional limitations and disability. Impairments noted include those associated with age and those specific to OA pathology. More work has been done on knee OA; increased pain, decreased range of motion, joint laxity, and decreased position sense have been identified as significant predictors.

Comorbidity

Verbrugge and colleagues[21] and Merikangas and colleagues[24] found that the effect of arthritis on functional limitations and disability was strongly increased in those who had other chronic conditions. Merikangas and colleagues[24] found that coefficients for regression models adjusting for comorbidity were decreased by one-half. Song and colleagues[8] also estimated that 20% of the excess risk for new disability in performing ADL related to arthritis could be attributed to the presence of comorbid conditions, and Ayis and colleagues[40] estimated an odds ratio of 3.6 for those with 3 or more comorbidities in their study of adults with lower extremity pain. Further studies support the important role of comorbidities in the development and progression of disability.[2,12,13,15,41]

Because OA is strongly associated with age, many with OA have comorbidities, and therefore understanding the specific contribution of arthritis, comorbidities, and related modifiable factors offers important opportunities to intervene. In particular, based on the evidence to date, interventions to decrease the risk of development of, for example, cardiac disease, obesity, depression, and stroke, would have more than an additive effect on future disability.

Obesity

Among others, several studies reviewed here have shown that overweight and obesity are not only a risk factor for OA, but also have direct and indirect effects on the progression of functional limitations and disability.[7,8,15,22,34,41] Mallen and colleagues[12] conducted a study to determine prognostic factors for functional limitations and disability for persons with knee pain and OA. One of the 4 generic indicators identified was body mass index (calculated as weight in kilograms divided by the square of height in meters). OA studies such as those described later in this article have begun to investigate the relationships among other factors, OA, disability, and obesity.

Self-efficacy

Self-efficacy has been identified as a factor mediating the relationship between knee pain, OA, and functional decline. In a longitudinal study of older adults with knee pain, low self-efficacy was a significant predictor of decline in stair climbing and self-reported physical function and disability (eg, taking care of a family member and shopping) for those with low baseline knee strength.[42] Other studies have shown the predictive nature of self-efficacy among adults with knee OA[14] and adults with knee OA and obesity.[43] Pells and colleagues[44] provided further evidence for the role of self-efficacy among overweight and obese adults with knee OA, and found that the role of self-efficacy depends on the specific aspect of OA examined. For example, self-efficacy for physical function was more strongly related to disability, and self-efficacy for pain was strongly related to reports of pain. Additional analyses were conducted to examine the relationship between self-efficacy for restraint in eating and actual restraint. This relationship was stronger than those for domain-specific self-efficacy related to pain and function. Using structural equation modeling, investigators have identified an additional variable, resilience, which has an indirect effect on pain, through self-efficacy.[45]

Psychosocial factors

The effect of psychological and social factors has been studied more extensively for knee OA than for OA involving other joints. However, as discussed earlier, in a model developed to identify prognostic indicators for functional outcome among those with knee pain and OA, anxiety was 1 of the 4 indicators.[12] Machado and colleagues,[39] reporting on results of 18-month follow-up with adults with physician-diagnosed OA, found that depressive symptoms mediated the relationship between symptoms and functional limitations and disability. Lamb and colleagues[34] investigated the relationship between knee pain and walking speed and ability to rise from a chair among participants in the Women's Health & Aging study with knee pain. In this cross-sectional study they found that depression modified the relationship between knee pain and functional mobility.

Larger studies using the broader definition of arthritis concur with studies focused on OA. Song and colleagues[8] found that depressive symptoms were significantly associated with functional limitations and disability in their longitudinal study of older adults with arthritis. Additional studies have demonstrated that depression exerts an important influence on disability in large national studies of those with arthritis.[24,31]

Parmelee and colleagues[46] investigated the relationship between depression, pain, functional limitation, and disability, modeling depressive symptoms as the outcome in a sample of persons with knee OA. Using linear and ordinary least squares regression analysis to develop path models of the associations between the variables, the investigators reported that pain was the main driver of the relationship between functional limitations and depressive symptoms. However, this was not the case for the relationships among pain, depressive symptoms, and disability; pain and disability predicted depressive symptoms.[46] This study provided evidence that participation in desired activities is associated with decreased depressive symptoms.

Level of exercise

Recent studies have found that exercise level is associated with functional limitations and disability, with aerobic and vigorous exercise providing a protective effect.[8,14,15,31]

Extra-individual Risk Factors

Two studies by Verbrugge and colleagues[25] addressed factors affecting the development of functional limitation or disability for those with arthritis using the National Health Interview Survey Disability Supplement, and were discussed briefly earlier in relation to other factors. The results of the first study indicated that persons with arthritis use more mobility aids, and fewer accommodations and assistance. Building on earlier work, Verbrugge and Juarez[9] explored buffers and barriers in a comparison of those with and without arthritis using Phase II of the Disability Supplement and compared persons with disabilities primarily caused by arthritis and those with disabilities primarily caused by other conditions. Arthritis-disabled persons reported more functional limitations, more buffers (medical devices and services, assistive equipment, and accommodations), and more barriers to getting around within and outside the home. Similar results were reported in a comparison of arthritis disability with heart disease disability using the same data source.[47] In addition, Wilkie and colleagues[33] showed that environmental factors such as need of aids and assistance, limited access to public transportation, and limited access to a car were predictive of disability.

Knowledge Gaps and Future Directions

One of the major limitations of the many studies of OA and its effect on disablement is the inclusion of risk factors cross-sectionally at baseline and the adjustment for these factors in analytical models. Most previous disablement research relies on single-equation systems in which hypothesized causes of disability are simultaneously entered into the analysis model to determine their effects on disability. Although this approach addresses the question of the effect or association of the pathology of OA and its relationship with subsequent functional limitations or disability outcomes, it has limited ability to elucidate the specific roles of the range of relevant risk or intervening factors that affect the progression of the disablement process across the continuum from pathology to disability, beyond and back through feedback loops. Future disablement research must clarify the causal mechanisms behind a potential risk factor's effect on disability and delineate the interplay between and among the various hypothesized steps in the disablement process. To know the extent with which OA is associated with functional loss and disability is important; to understand the critical factors that mediate these associations is crucial if we are to design evidence-based interventions aimed at retarding or preventing the disablement process for those with OA.

Lawrence and Jette[48] provide an example of 1 alternative analytical approach in their investigation of the relationship between risk factors, impairments, functional limitations, and disability using data from a cohort of older adults. They used the Disablement Model as the conceptual model for the causal mechanisms involved, and structural equation modeling to test the hypotheses generated by the model. Their modeling underscored the important intervening role of lower extremity function in protecting against the subsequent onset of disability and revealed the significant buffering role played by level of physical activity in the onset of future functional limitations and disability. Machado and colleagues[39] also applied a hypothesized model of the relationship between impairment (symptom severity), and disability divided into activity limitations and participation restrictions specific to OA. They used exploratory factor analysis to test their hypothesis that physical symptoms effect higher level disability through lower level physical functional limitations and depressive symptoms. Results supported this hypothesis, indicating that symptom severity causes limitations in specific functional tasks and depressive symptoms, and that persons with these limitations in turn limit their participation in social roles and activities. The investigators posited that the subsequent limitations could be because social roles and activities actually include these specific physical functions within their larger, more complex activities and that the depressive symptoms in turn cause limitations in the ability or desire to take part in social roles and activities. In providing detail for the causal mechanisms and relative contributions of physical symptoms and functional limitations, their results make an important contribution to understanding the disablement process in OA.

Although there are many opportunities to improve our understanding of the specific role of risk factors, intra-individual factors, and extra-individual factors in the relationships among pathology, impairment, functional limitations, and disability, the analytical models used need to be consistent with the objectives of this disablement research. The authors have highlighted 2 examples of potential approaches to advancing our understanding of these factors. There are others in the OA literature; for example, the use of ordinary least squares regression to model pathways.[46] However, for most factors discussed, the temporal pattern and relative impacts on key disability milestones are relatively unknown. Future work should use longitudinal data to test hypotheses about the relative effect of these factors rather than adjusting for them.

REFERENCES

1. Covinsky K. Aging, arthritis, and disability. Arthritis Rheum 2006;55(2):175–6.
2. Covinsky KE, Lindquist K, Dunlop DD, et al. Effect of arthritis in middle age on older-age functioning. J Am Geriatr Soc 2008;56(1):23–8.
3. Dunlop D, Hughes S, Manheim L. Disability in activities of daily living: patterns of change and a hierarchy of disability. Am J Public Health 1997;87:378–83.
4. Dunlop D, Manheim L, Song J, et al. Arthritis prevalence and activity limitations in older adults. Arthritis Rheum 2001;44(1):212–21.
5. Felson D, Lawrence R, Dieppe P, et al. Osteoarthritis: new insights. Part 1: the disease and its risk factors [review]. Ann Intern Med 2000;133(8):635–46.
6. Institute of Medicine (IOM). The future of disability in America. Washington, DC: The National Academies Press; 2007.
7. Ling SM, Xue QL, Simonsick EM, et al. Transitions to mobility difficulty associated with lower extremity osteoarthritis in high functioning older women: longitudinal data from the Women's Health and Aging Study II. Arthritis Rheum 2006;55(2): 256–63.
8. Song J, Chang RW, Dunlop DD. Population impact of arthritis on disability in older adults. Arthritis Rheum 2006;55(2):248–55.
9. Verbrugge LM, Juarez L. Profile of arthritis disability: II. Arthritis Rheum 2006; 55(1):102–13.
10. van Saase JL, van Romunde L, Cats A, et al. Epidemiology of arthritis: Zoetermeer survey. Comparison of radiological arthritis in a Dutch population with that of 10 other populations. Ann Rheum Dis 1989;20:351–69.
11. Ferrucci L, Guralnik JM, Simonsick E, et al. Progressive versus catastrophic disability: a longitudinal view of the disablement process. J Gerontol A Biol Sci Med Sci 1996;51(3):M123–30.
12. Mallen CD, Peat G, Thomas E, et al. Predicting poor functional outcome in community-dwelling older adults with knee pain: prognostic value of generic indicators. Ann Rheum Dis 2007;66(11):1456–61.
13. Roos EM, Bremander AB, Englund M, et al. Change in self-reported outcomes and objective physical function over 7 years in middle-aged subjects with or at high risk of knee osteoarthritis. Ann Rheum Dis 2008;67(4):505–10.

14. Sharma L, Cahue S, Song J, et al. Physical functioning over three years in knee osteoarthritis: role of psychosocial, local mechanical, and neuromuscular factors. Arthritis Rheum 2003;48(12):3359–70.

15. van Dijk GM, Dekker J, Veenhof C, et al. Course of functional status and pain in osteoarthritis of the hip or knee: a systematic review of the literature. Arthritis Rheum 2006;55(5):779–85.

16. Lawrence J, Bremner JM, Bier F. Prevalence in the population and relationships between symptoms and x-ray changes. Ann Rheum Dis 1966; 25:1–24.

17. Jette A. Disentangling the process of disablement. Soc Sci Med 1999;48:471–2.

18. Nagi S. Some conceptual issues disability and rehabilitation. In: Sussman M, editor. Sociology and rehabilitation. Washington, DC: American Sociology Association; 1965. p. 100–13.

19. Nagi S. The concept and measurement of disability. In: Berkowitz ED, editor. Disability policies and government programs. New York: Praeger; 1979.

20. Verbrugge LM, Jette AM. The disablement process. Soc Sci Med 1994;38(1):1–14.

21. Verbrugge LM, Lepkowski JM, Konkol LL, et al. Levels of disability among U.S. adults with arthritis. J Gerontol 1991;46(2):S71–83.

22. Verbrugge LM, Gates DM, Ike RW, et al. Risk factors for disability among U.S. adults with arthritis. J Clin Epidemiol 1991;44(2):167–82.

23. Hochberg MC, Kasper J, Williamson J, et al. The contribution of osteoarthritis to disability: preliminary data from the Women's Health and Aging Study. J Rheumatol Suppl 1995;43:16–8.

24. Merikangas K, Ames M, Cui L, et al. The impact of comorbidity of mental and physical conditions on role disability in the US adult household population. Arch Gen Psychiatry 2007;64(10):1180–8.

25. Verbrugge LM, Juarez L, Verbrugge LM, et al. Profile of arthritis disability. Public Health Rep 2001;116(Suppl 1):157–79.

26. Guccione A, Felson D, Anderson J, et al. The effects of specific medical conditions on the functional limitations of elders in the Framingham Study. Am J Public Health 1994;84(3):351–8.

27. Reginster JY, Khaltaev NG, Reginster JY, et al. Introduction and WHO perspective on the global burden of musculoskeletal conditions. Rheumatology (Oxford) 2002;41(Supp 1):1–2.

28. Fautrel B, Hilliquin P, Rozenberg S, et al. Impact of osteoarthritis: results of a nationwide survey of 10,000 patients consulting for OA. Joint Bone Spine 2005;72(3):235–40.

29. Zhang Y, Niu J, Kally-Hayes M, et al. Prevalence of symptomatic hand osteoarthritis and its impact on functional status among the elderly. Am J Epidemiol 2002;156:1021–7.

30. Dekker J, van Dijk GM, Veenhof C, et al. Risk factors for functional decline in osteoarthritis of the hip or knee. Curr Opin Rheumatol 2009;21(5):520–4.

31. Dunlop DD, Semanik P, Song J, et al. Risk factors for functional decline in older adults with arthritis. Arthritis Rheum 2005;52(4):1274–82.

32. Wilkie R, Peat G, Thomas E, et al. Factors associated with participation restriction in community-dwelling adults aged 50 years and over. Qual Life Res 2007;16(7):1147–56.

33. Wilkie R, Peat G, Thomas E, et al. Factors associated with restricted mobility outside the home in community-dwelling adults ages fifty years and older with knee pain: an example of use of the international classification of functioning to investigate participation restriction. Arthritis Rheum 2007;57(8): 1381–9.

34. Lamb SE, Guralnik JM, Buchner DM, et al. Factors that modify the association between knee pain and mobility limitation in older women: the Women's Health and Aging Study. Ann Rheum Dis 2000;59(5):331–7.
35. Mottram S, Peat G, Thomas E, et al. Patterns of pain and mobility limitation in older people: cross-sectional findings from a population survey of 18,497 adults aged 50 years and over. Qual Life Res 2008;17(4):529–39.
36. van Dijk GM, Veenhof C, Spreeuwenberg P, et al. Prognosis of limitations in activities in osteoarthritis of the hip or knee: a 3-year cohort study. Arch Phys Med Rehabil 2010;91(1):58–66.
37. Miller ME, Rejeski WJ, Messier SP, et al. Modifiers of change in physical functioning in older adults with knee pain: the Observational Arthritis Study in Seniors (OASIS). Arthritis Rheum 2001;45(4):331–9.
38. Jinks C, Jordan K, Croft P, et al. Osteoarthritis as a public health problem: the impact of developing knee pain on physical function in adults living in the community: (KNEST 3). Rheumatology (Oxford) 2007;46(5):877–81.
39. Machado GP, Gignac MA, Badley EM, et al. Participation restrictions among older adults with osteoarthritis: a mediated model of physical symptoms, activity limitations, and depression. Arthritis Rheum 2008;59(1):129–35.
40. Ayis S, Dieppe P, Ayis S, et al. The natural history of disability and its determinants in adults with lower limb musculoskeletal pain. J Rheumatol 2009;36(3):583–91.
41. Peters TJ, Sanders C, Dieppe P, et al. Factors associated with change in pain and disability over time: a community-based prospective observational study of hip and knee osteoarthritis. Br J Gen Pract 2005;55(512):205–11.
42. Rejeski WJ, Miller ME, Foy C, et al. Self-efficacy and the progression of functional limitations and self-reported disability in older adults with knee pain. J Gerontol B Psychol Sci Soc Sci 2001;56(5):S261–5.
43. Shelby RA, Somers TJ, Keefe FJ, et al. Domain specific self-efficacy mediates the impact of pain catastrophizing on pain and disability in overweight and obese osteoarthritis patients. J Pain 2008;9(10):912–9.
44. Pells JJ, Shelby RA, Keefe FJ, et al. Arthritis self-efficacy and self-efficacy for resisting eating: relationships to pain, disability, and eating behavior in overweight and obese individuals with osteoarthritic knee pain. Pain 2008;136(3):340–7.
45. Wright LJ, Zautra AJ, Going S, et al. Adaptation to early knee osteoarthritis: the role of risk, resilience, and disease severity on pain and physical functioning. Ann Behav Med 2008;36(1):70–80.
46. Parmelee P, Harralson T, Smith L, et al. Necessary and discretionary activities in knee osteoarthritis: do they mediate the pain-depression relationship? Pain Med 2007;8(5):449–61.
47. Verbrugge LM, Juarez L, Verbrugge LM, et al. Arthritis disability and heart disease disability. Arthritis Rheum 2008;59(10):1445–57.
48. Lawrence RH, Jette AM. Disentangling the disablement process. J Gerontol B Psychol Sci Soc Sci 1996;51(4):S173–82.

Quality of Osteoarthritis Care for Community-Dwelling Older Adults

David J. Hunter, MBBS, PhD, FRACP[a,b,*]

KEYWORDS

• Osteoarthritis • Clinical care • Health care quality
• Older adults

Osteoarthritis is a rising epidemic. In 2000, there were 25 million north Americans with osteoarthritis (OA).[1,2] By 2020, the number of people with OA will have doubled, in large part because of the exploding prevalence of obesity and the graying of the baby boomer generation. The largest increases will occur among older adults, for whom OA also has the greatest functional impact. Despite growing concern, OA remains a poorly understood disease and recent doubts about the safety of several commonly prescribed OA medications have served to highlight deficiencies in the traditional medical approach to management. Current clinical management for OA is often limited to analgesic medication and cautious waiting[3] for the sometimes eventual referral for total joint replacement. With few conservative options offered by their doctors, increasing numbers of patients are turning to untested folk remedies and aggressively marketed dietary supplements with little substantive evidence to support their efficacy.

There is great demand for non-pharmacologic therapies and a pressing need for clinicians to revisit the quality of their current clinical management for OA. What follows is a general outline for the management of patients with OA, how standard clinical practice diverges from what is recommended, some key challenges facing clinicians with regards optimizing quality of care delivery in OA, and steps to improve

Dr Hunter is funded by an Australian Research Council Future Fellowship.
Conflict of interest statement: The corresponding author had full access to all the data in the study and had final responsibility for the decision to submit for publication. Dr Hunter receives research or institutional support from AstraZeneca, DonJoy, Lilly, Merck, NIH, Pfizer, Stryker, and Wyeth.
[a] Department of Rheumatology, Northern Clinical School, University of Sydney, 2065, Sydney, Australia
[b] Division of Research, New England Baptist Hospital, 125 Parker Hill Avenue, Boston, MA 02120, USA
* Rheumatology Department, Level 4, Block 4, Royal North Shore Hospital, St Leonards 2065, New South Wales, Australia.
E-mail address: David.Hunter@sydney.edu.au

the OA health care quality in the form of a narrative review. For the interested clinician further references are provided that can facilitate additional reading and hopefully practice change.[4-9] Inevitably there is much the interested clinician can do rather than nihilistic waiting. The author encourages active clinician involvement, instilling much of what are self-management strategies in their patients, and optimizing the evidence-based nature of practice and the quality of care to further promote more effective long-term treatment of this pervasive disease.

THE PUBLIC HEALTH BURDEN OF OSTEOARTHRITIS

Recent estimates suggest that symptomatic knee OA occurs in 13% of individuals aged 60 years and older.[10,11] The risk for mobility disability (defined as needing help walking or climbing stairs) attributable to knee OA alone is greater than that caused by any other medical condition in people aged 65 years and older.[12,13] Although this prevalence is high, it is expected to increase even further with the obesity epidemic and aging baby-boomer population.[14]

In addition to its societal impact, the burden of knee OA can be measured by its impact on quality of life. OA was estimated to be the eighth leading cause of non-fatal burden in the world in 1990, accounting for 2.8% of total years lost because of disease (YLD), around the same percentage as schizophrenia and congenital anomalies.[15] In the Version 2 estimates for the Global Burden of Disease 2000 study, published in the World Health Report 2002,[16] OA is the fourth leading cause of YLDs at the global level.

The United States spends more than $2.2 trillion nationally on health care each year, equal to16% of the gross domestic product (GDP). Health care spending is projected to increase to $4 trillion by 2017, which is almost 20% of the economy. This continued growth is not sustainable and has been responsible in part for recent calls for health care reform. The major platforms of health care control will be cost containment through optimizing effectiveness and quality.

One of the most expensive aspects of health care delivery is management of osteoarthritis. According to the US Centers for Disease Control, arthritis and other rheumatic conditions cost the United States $128 billion in 2003, a 24% surge since 1997 and an amount equal to 1.2% of the GDP.[17] The most prevalent and disabling form of arthritis is osteoarthritis.

OSTEOARTHRITIS MANAGEMENT

The management goals for patients with osteoarthritis are

- Patient education about the disease and its management
- Pain control
- Improve function and decrease disability
- Alter the disease process and its consequences.

In the absence of a cure, current therapeutic modalities are primarily aimed at reducing pain and improving joint function by modalities targeted toward symptom relief that do not facilitate any improvement in joint structure. The management of OA should be individualized so that it conforms to the specific findings of the clinical examination. This individualization is especially important for findings of obesity, malalignment, and muscle weakness. Comprehensive management always includes a combination of treatment options that are directed towards the common goal of improving patients' pain and tolerance for functional activity. Treatment plans should never be defined rigidly according to the radiographic appearance of the joint, but should instead remain flexible so that they can be altered according to the functional and symptomatic responses obtained.

The recommended hierarchy of management should consist of non-pharmacologic modalities first, drugs, and then surgery. Too frequently the first step is forgotten or not emphasized sufficiently to the patients' detriment.[3] In addition, combinations of treatments are frequently used in clinical practice and may have additional synergistic benefits.

There are several available well-written guidelines that describe the management of osteoarthritis that are based on evidence from trials and expert consensus.[4-7]

PLETHORA OF GUIDELINES

Recent years have seen several evidence-based guidelines developed for osteoarthritis management,[4-9] including the most recent additions from the Osteoarthritis Research Society International (OARSI) and the American Academy of Orthopaedic Surgeons (AAOS). There is some consistency[18-20] in the numerous guidelines that are available for OA management,[4-9] yet despite some dissemination attempts, clinical practice does not reflect these recommendations.[3,20-22] **Table 1** depicts the recommendations that were developed by the OARSI Treatment Guidelines Committee.[7] These recommendations emanated from a combined evidence consensus approach and have been widely endorsed by clinicians, professional groups, and some payers. This committee undertook a critical appraisal of published guidelines and a systematic review of more recent evidence for relevant therapies and was completed and published in two parts in late 2007 and early 2008. The recommendations represent an overarching grouping of non-pharmacologic conservative interventions, pharmacologic and surgical interventions that are consistent with recommendations that conservative, safer interventions be adopted prior to interventions with more adverse safety and cost profiles. The recommendations are summarized in **Table 1** together with the level of research evidence supporting them; the effect size for pain relief (ES_{pain} [95% CI]); the extent of consensus (%); and the strength of recommendation (mean+/- standard error of the mean) for each proposition. The recommendations are broadly consistent regarding the content of other guideline recommendations. Despite the consistency and the number of guidelines that are available to practicing clinicians, there is a divergence of what is recommended to clinicians and what occurs in clinical practice.[3,20-22] The remainder of this article focuses upon what commonly happens in clinical practice, interventions that should be more commonly practiced, and measures that can be taken to overcome this divergence.

CLINICAL PRACTICE DOES NOT REFLECT WHAT IS RECOMMENDED

In the absence of a cure, current therapeutic modalities are primarily aimed at reducing pain and improving joint function primarily using agents targeted toward symptoms that do not facilitate any improvement in joint structure or long-term disease amelioration.[4-9] The most widely used agents, nonsteroidal antiinflammatory drugs (NSAIDs) and cyclooxygenase 2 (COX-2) inhibitors, are associated with high rates of adverse events.[23,24] NSAIDs alone cause over 16,500 deaths and over 103,000 hospitalizations per year in the United States.[25] In addition, these drugs rarely relieve symptoms completely. In clinical trials of OA, different NSAIDs performed similarly, with subjects reporting an approximate 30% reduction in pain and 15% improvement in function.[26]

Table 1
OARSI recommendations and research evidence

Proposition	Level of Evidence	Effect Size for Pain (95% CI)	Frequency Recommended in Existing Guidelines	Level of Consensus (%)	Strength of Recommendation (% [95% CI])
General					
1. Optimal management of OA requires a combination of non-pharmacological and pharmacological modalities.	IV	—	12/12	100%	96 (93–99)
Non-pharmacological modalities of treatment					
2. All patients with hip and knee OA should be given information access and education about the objectives of treatment and the importance of changes in lifestyle, exercise, pacing of activities, weight reduction, and other measures to unload the damaged joints. The initial focus should be on self-help and patient-driven treatments rather than on passive therapies delivered by health professionals. Subsequently, emphasis should be placed on encouraging adherence to the regimen of non-pharmacological therapy.	Ia (education) IV (adherence)	0.06 (0.02, 0.10)	8/8	92%	97 (95–99)
3. The clinical status of patients with hip or knee OA can be improved if patients are contacted regularly by phone.	Ia	0.12 (0.00, 0.24)	2/2	77%	66 (57–75)
4. Patients with symptomatic hip and knee OA may benefit from referral to a physical therapist for evaluation and instruction in appropriate exercises to reduce pain and improve functional capacity. This evaluation may result in provision of assistive devices, such as canes and walkers, as appropriate.	IV	—	5/5	100%	89 (82–96)
5. Patients with hip and knee OA should be encouraged to undertake, and continue to undertake, regular aerobic, muscle-strengthening, and range- of -motion exercises. For patients with symptomatic hip OA, exercises in water can be effective.	Ia (knee) IV(hip) Ib (hip, water-based)	0.52 (0.34, 0.70) aerobic 0.32 (0.23, 0.42) strength 0.25 (0.02, 0.47) water based	21/21 21/21 8/8	85%	96 (93–99)

#	Recommendation					
6.	Patients with hip and knee OA, who are overweight, should be encouraged to lose weight and maintain their weight at a lower level.	Ia	0.13 (-0.12, 0.38)	13/14	100%	96 (92–100)
7.	Walking aids can reduce pain in patients with hip and knee OA. Patients should be given instruction in the optimal use of a cane or crutch in the contralateral hand. Frames or wheeled walkers are often preferable for those with bilateral disease.	IV	—	11/11	100%	90 (84–96)
8.	In patients with knee OA and mild/moderate varus or valgus instability, a knee brace can reduce pain, improve stability and diminish the risk of falling.	Ia	—	8/9	92%	76 (69–83)
9.	Every patient with hip or knee OA should receive advice concerning appropriate footwear. In patients with knee OA insoles can reduce pain and improve ambulation. Lateral wedged insoles can be of symptomatic benefit for some patients with medial tibiofemoral compartment OA.	IV (footwear) Ia (insole)	—	12/13	92%	77 (66–88)
10.	Some thermal modalities may be effective for relieving symptoms in hip and knee OA.	Ia	0.69 (-0.07, 1.45)	7/10	77%	64 (60–68)
11.	Transcutaneous electrical nerve stimulation can help with short-term pain control in some patients with hip or knee OA.	Ia	—	8/10	69%	58 (45–72)
12.	Acupuncture may be of symptomatic benefit in patients with knee OA.	Ia	0.51 (0.23, 0.79)	5/8	69%	59 (47–71)

Pharmacological modalities of treatment

#	Recommendation					
13.	Acetaminophen (up to 4 g/d) can be an effective initial oral analgesic for treatment of mild to moderate pain in patients with knee or hip OA. In the absence of an adequate response, or in the presence of severe pain or inflammation, alternative pharmacologic therapy should be considered based on relative efficacy and safety, and concomitant medications and comorbidities.	Ia (knee) IV (hip)	0.21 (0.02, 0.41)	16/16	77%	92 (88–99)

(continued on next page)

Table 1
(continued)

Proposition	Level of Evidence	Effect Size for Pain (95% CI)	Frequency Recommended in Existing Guidelines	Level of Consensus (%)	Strength of Recommendation (% [95% CI])
14. In patients with symptomatic hip or knee OA, NSAIDs should be used at the lowest effective dose but their long-term use should be avoided if possible. In patients with increased gastrointestinal risk, either a COX-2 selective agent or a non-selective NSAID with co-prescription of a proton pump inhibitor or misoprostol for gastroprotection may be considered, but NSAIDs, including non-selective and COX-2 selective agents, should be used with caution in patients with cardiovascular risk factors.	Ia (knee) Ia (hip)	0.32 (0.24, 0.39)	NSAID + PPi 8/8 NSAID + misoprostol 8/8 COX-2 inhibitors 11/11	100%	93 (88–99)
15. Topical NSAIDs and capsaicin can be effective as adjunctives and alternatives to oral analgesic/antiinflammatory agents in knee OA.	Ia (NSAIDs) Ia (capsaicin)	0.41 (0.22, 0.59)	7/9 8/9	100%	85 (75–95)
16. IA injections with corticosteroids can be used in the treatment of hip or knee OA, and should be considered particularly when patients have moderate to severe pain not responding satisfactorily to oral analgesic/antiinflammatory agents and in patients with symptomatic knee OA with effusions or other physical signs of local inflammation.	Ib (hip) Ia (knee)	0.72 (0.42, 1.02)	11/13	69%	78 (61–95)
17. Injections of intraarticular hyaluronate may be useful in patients with knee or hip OA. They are characterized by delayed onset, but prolonged duration, of symptomatic benefit when compared to IA injections of corticosteroids.	Ia (knee) Ia (hip)	0.32 (0.17, 0.47)	8/9	85%	64 (43–85)
18. Treatment with glucosamine or chondroitin sulfate may provide symptomatic benefit in patients with knee OA. If no response is apparent within 6 months treatment should be discontinued.	Ia (glucosamine) Ia (chondroitin)	0.45 (0.04, 0.86) 0.30 (−0.10, 0.70)	6/10 2/7	92%	63 (44–82)

No.	Recommendation	Level of evidence		%	CI
19.	In patients with symptomatic knee OA, glucosamine sulfate and chondroitin sulfate may have structure-modifying effects, whereas diacerein may have structure-modifying effects in patients with symptomatic OA of the hip.	Ib (knee) Ib (hip)	—	69%	41 (20–62)
20.	The use of weak opioids and narcotic analgesics can be considered for the treatment of refractory pain in patients with hip or knee OA where other pharmacological agents have been ineffective, or are contraindicated. Stronger opioids should only be used for the management of severe pain in exceptional circumstances. Non-pharmacological therapies should be continued in such patients and surgical treatments should be considered.	Ia (week opioids) IV (strong opioids) IV (others)	9/9	92%	82 (74–90)
	Surgical modalities of treatment				
21.	Patients with hip or knee OA who are not obtaining adequate pain relief and functional improvement from a combination of non-pharmacological and pharmacological treatment should be considered for joint replacement surgery. Replacement arthroplasties are effective and cost-effective interventions for patients with significant symptoms or functional limitations associated with a reduced health-related quality of life, despite conservative therapy.	III	14/14	92%	96 (94–98)
22.	Unicompartmental knee replacement is effective in patients with knee OA restricted to a single compartment.	IIb	—	100%	76 (64–88)
23.	Osteotomy and joint preserving surgical procedures should be considered in young adults with symptomatic hip OA, especially in the presence of dysplasia. For young and physically active patients with significant symptoms from unicompartmental knee OA, high tibial osteotomy may offer an alternative intervention that delays the need for joint replacement for approximately 10 years.	IIb	10/10	100%	75 (64–86)

(continued on next page)

Table 1
(continued)

Proposition	Level of Evidence	Effect Size for Pain (95% CI)	Frequency Recommended in Existing Guidelines	Level of Consensus (%)	Strength of Recommendation (% [95% CI])
24. The role of joint lavage and arthroscopic debridement in knee OA are controversial. Although some studies have demonstrated short-term symptom relief, others suggest that improvement in symptoms could be attributable to a placebo effect.	Ib (lavage) Ib (debridement)	0.09 (-0.27, 0.44) -0.01(-0.37, 0.35)	3/3 5/6	100%	60 (47–82)
25. In patients with OA of the knee, joint fusion can be considered as a salvage procedure when joint replacement has failed.	IV	—	2/2	100%	69 (57–82)

Level of evidence: Ia, meta-analysis of randomized controlled trials; Ib, randomized controlled trial; IIa, controlled study without randomization; IIb, quasi-experimental study (eg, uncontrolled trial, one arm dose-response trial, and so forth); III, observational studies (eg, case-control, cohort, cross-sectional studies); IV, expert opinion.

Effect size is the standard mean difference (ie, the mean difference between a treatment and a control group divided by the standard deviation of the difference). ES of 0.2 is considered small, ES of 0.5 is moderate, and ES greater than 0.8 is large.

Abbreviations: COX-2, cyclooxygenase 2; ES, effect size; IA, intraarticular; IV, intravenous; NSAID, non-steroidal anti inflammatory analgesic drug; RCT, randomized controlled trial.

From Zhang W, Moskovitz R, Nuki G, et al. OARSI recommendations for the management of hip and knee osteoarthritis, part II: OARSI evidence-based, expert consensus guidelines. Osteoarthritis Cartilage 2008;16:137–62; with permission.

Many individuals with OA ultimately require total joint replacement, a procedure that is also not without inherent morbidity and cost. Although osteoarthritis can be treated surgically, there are many patients for whom this is inappropriate because of medical comorbidity, old age, or other circumstances.[7] In the younger and more active individual, it is desirable to delay arthroplasty because of the limited lifespan of the prosthesis and the necessary lifestyle changes that accompany it.

With few conservative options offered by their doctors, increasing numbers of patients are turning to untested folk remedies and aggressively marketed dietary supplements with little substantive evidence to support their efficacy.[27] Despite several evidence-based guidelines for OA management,[4–9] several reports have outlined suboptimal care for patients with OA.[3,20–22]

There are just a few of the major current challenges in OA management that reflect a divergence from what is recommended in evidence-based guidelines. Areas for divergence from quality care include inadequate uptake of conservative, non-pharmacologic treatment options, such as weight loss and exercise; inappropriate surgical interventions, such as arthroscopic debridement and lavage in the absence of mechanical disturbance in the knee; increasing volume of arthroplasty surgery that is not sustainable; and the inappropriate use of imaging. These are just a few of the examples that are discussed further here, but inevitably the challenges need to be ascertained and endorsed by the interested stakeholders (including clinicians engaged in OA management).

Obesity Management

The majority of patients with arthritis are either overweight or obese. There is good evidence for the efficacy of weight management,[28] and this is advocated by most OA guidelines. However, in practice, weight management is not frequently implemented.[21,29,30]

Exercise

Another pivotal and frequently ignored[21,29,30] aspect of conservative treatment of OA is exercise. Exercise increases aerobic capacity, muscle strength, and endurance, and also facilitates weight loss.[28,31] All individuals capable of exercise should be encouraged to partake in a low-impact aerobic exercise program (walking, biking, swimming, or other aquatic exercise). Quadricep strengthening exercises have been demonstrated to lead to improvements in pain and function.[32–34] Guidelines routinely advocate exercise,[4–9] however, clinical practice does not reflect this recommendation.[21,29,30]

Surgical Challenges

Surgery should be resisted when symptoms can be managed by other treatment modalities. At present there is no metric whereby the use of conservative management prior to surgery is monitored. The typical indications for surgery are debilitating pain and major limitation of functions, such as walking, working, or sleeping.[35] Although joint replacement has a large effect size,[36–38] it is an invasive treatment that has attendant risks. If surgical intervention is to be pursued, recent evidence has shown that patients operated upon in low-volume hospitals or by low-volume surgeons have worse functional outcomes 2 years post total knee replacement than those operated upon in high-volume hospitals by high-volume surgeons.[39] However, surgical funding and resources are not necessarily linked to optimizing outcomes and reducing risk. In addition, several studies have suggested that up to 30% of some surgical procedures are inappropriate.[40,41] Eliminating inappropriate surgery has the potential to contain rising costs.

Two of the main surgical challenges in quality improvement are: (1) The most common orthopedic procedure (arthroscopic debridement and lavage) is ineffective. (2) The demand for joint replacement is increasing faster than surgeon supply and health care costs can sustain, and rational ways of optimizing treatment for those who receive joint replacement may be required.

Arthroscopic debridement and lavage

The most common orthopedic surgery performed on the knee has no demonstrable efficacy.[42] Arthroscopic debridement and meniscal resection remains the most frequently performed procedure by orthopedic surgeons in the United States,[43,44] with up to 1 million knee arthroscopies performed annually in the United States. The majority of these procedures appear to be performed for a meniscal tear in older individuals with underlying OA and superimposed degenerative meniscal tears. The lack of a comprehensive ambulatory surgery database in the United States precludes more precise estimates of arthroscopy utilization.

Degenerative meniscal lesions, such as horizontal cleavages and oblique or complex tears, are associated with older age.[45] By the time radiographic disease develops, the overwhelming majority of individuals have meniscal lesions.[45,46] In asymptomatic subjects with a mean age of 65 years, a tear was found in 67% using MRI, whereas in patients with symptomatic knee OA, a meniscal tear was found in 91%.[46] Resection of a nonobstructive degenerate meniscus may only remove the earliest evidence of this disorder while the OA degradation proceeds.[42]

In a well-designed placebo surgery trial, improvement in symptoms could be attributed to a placebo effect.[42] For a subgroup of knees with loose bodies or flaps of meniscus or cartilage that are causing mechanical symptoms, especially locking or catching of the joint, arthroscopic removal of these unstable tissues may improve joint function and alleviate these mechanical symptoms. The majority of patients with knee OA do not complain of these symptoms. Recent guidelines, including those from OARSI and AAOS, recommend against the use of routine arthroscopy for knee OA management. To date these recommendations have not been reflected in changes in clinical practice.

Arthroplasty

The development of modern total hip arthroplasty in the 1960s by John Charnley, a British surgeon, represents a milestone in orthopedic surgery. Currently the most common indication for knee and hip replacement (approximately 85% of all cases) is OA. The general consensus among orthopedic surgeons on indicators for these operative procedures, carried out by a postal survey, were (1) severe daily pain and (2) radiographic evidence of joint space narrowing.[35] With proper patient selection, good to excellent results can be expected in 95% of patients, and the survival rate of the implant is expected to be 95% at 15 years.[47] When overall health improvement is used to assess the cost effectiveness of total joint arthroplasty, the hip and knee arthroplasty have similar results.[48]

The utilization of total knee replacement increased by more than 10% per year in the late 1980s and continues to climb, with more than 350,000 primary total knee replacement procedures and 29,000 revision procedures performed in the United States in 2002.[49] The common complications observed during the 90 days following primary knee replacement include mortality (0.7%); readmission (0.9%); pulmonary embolus

(0.8%); wound infection (0.4%); pneumonia (1.4%); and myocardial infarction (0.8%).[49]

Over the next decade, demand for arthroplasty is projected to increase dramatically. Substantial increases in the number of hip and knee replacement surgeries are predicted from 2005 to 2030.[50] Primary total hip arthroplasty is estimated to grow by 174%, from 208,600 in 2005 to 572,100 by 2030, whereas primary total knee arthroplasty is projected to grow from 450,400 to 3.48 million procedures during the same period (more than 673%).[50] The size of the orthopedic workforce is not positioned to cater for this increase in volume and the current state of the economy is unlikely able to withstand this continued increase in expenditure.

Imaging

Imaging can assist in making a diagnosis of OA by refuting other diagnoses when the clinical picture from history and physical examination leaves this diagnosis unclear.[51] The diagnosis is, however, a clinical one made by assessing the constellation of presenting clinical features and radiography should be used only to refute other diagnoses that could plausibly result in patients' symptoms. Currently there is an overuse of inappropriate imaging to make a diagnosis that can be made clinically. In light of the current lack of therapy that can modify the disease course and measurement imprecision, there is currently no rationale for obtaining serial radiographs if the clinical state remains unchanged. MRI should only be used in infrequent circumstances to facilitate the diagnosis of other causes of knee pain that can be confused with osteoarthritis (eg, osteochondritis dissecans, avascular necrosis). The presence of a meniscal tear viewed by MRI in a person with knee osteoarthritis is almost uniform and is not necessarily a cause of increased symptoms.[46] The penchant to remove menisci is to be avoided, unless there are symptoms of locking or extension blockade[52] because there is strong data to support that meniscectomy, even partial meniscectomy, increases the risk for progression of OA.[53]

Eliminating unproven procedures and reducing needless costs is necessary if the nation is to improve the quality and lower the cost of care over all. Various medical procedures in the United States, such as CT, MRI, and PET scans, have grown to a $100 billion industry in the United States, of which $14 billion has been shouldered by Medicare. According to Dr. Vijay Rao, chairwoman of the radiology department of the Thomas Jefferson University Hospital, of the more than 95 million high-tech scans done in the United States annually, 20% to 50% are unnecessary because their results failed to help treat or diagnose the patients' ailment.

FROM GUIDELINE RECOMMENDATIONS TO CLINICAL PRACTICE

Evidence-based guidelines have the potential to improve the quality of health care by promoting interventions of proven benefit and discouraging unnecessary, ineffective, or harmful interventions.[54] Given the number of guidelines available for OA, and the consistency of recommendations within them, and considering the time and resources required for guideline development, future efforts to guide management of OA of the hip or knee are better directed towards implementing practices known to be effective, and facilitating research to answer important questions where there is little evidence.[18]

There is worldwide interest in developing and implementing patient-centered models of care to support integration of evidence into practice and improve patient health outcomes for people with chronic conditions, including OA.[55,56]

The complex factors driving these health service reforms are well summarized in the Institute of Medicine (IOM) pivotal report, *Crossing the quality chasm: a new health system for the 21st century*, "there is... more to know, more to do, more to manage, more to watch and more people involved than ever before."[57]

The IOM report[58] defines 10 rules for system redesign to meet the needs of those with chronic conditions, one of which relates to evidence-based decision making. Patients should receive standardized care that is evidence based. Care should not vary illogically from clinician to clinician or from place to place.

OA management system redesign should consider all quality of care domains: that care is safe, effective, patient-centered, timely, efficient, and equitable.[59] The historical approach to the uptake of evidence into practice has been to focus on passive dissemination (diffusion) of information to individuals through social networks in which an assumption is made that the target individuals are aware, motivated, and capable of implementing necessary change. Support for this process has relied on the provision of resources in the form of standardized, evidence-based clinical practice guidelines and provision of skills training in the use of evidence-based medicine methods. Educational methods have involved use of passive continuous medical education methods.

Several papers document widespread support for OA guidelines, but there are delays in uptake, particularly of non-pharmacological recommendations, and variance in the application of recommendations by clinicians in different contexts.[21,22,60–62] In addition, qualitative information suggests that the needs of patients are not being met with regard to the quantity and quality of information provided about OA and its treatment, the emotional needs of patients, and patient-clinician communication.[63,64]

Three main issues that influence the use of evidence in medical care are quality of evidence, barriers and facilitators to practice change, and effective dissemination and implementation strategies.[65] Barriers to changing practice exist within patients, professionals, health care teams, healthcare organizations, and the wider environment.[23] Pencharz and colleagues evaluated six lower-limb OA guidelines, including the The European League Against Rheumatism (EULAR) and American College of Rheumatology (ACR) guidelines, and found that almost none of them addressed implementation strategies and barriers to use of the guidelines.[20] In general, few guidelines are evaluated for effectiveness of dissemination strategies and even fewer for the health impact of the guideline.[66]

Future research should be directed towards overcoming patient and provider barriers to the use of OA guidelines and their documentation, guideline implementation, and evaluation of outcomes. Although the evidence for many OA treatments is good, the complexity and high number of treatment recommendations available for OA may be a hindrance to use of the guidelines. Many strategies have been evaluated to improve implementation of evidence into practice.

Grimshaw and colleagues, in their systematic review of strategies, found that there was no magic bullet to promote implementation; however, generally effective strategies include financial interventions for clinicians (compensation hitched to quality metrics), reminder systems, interactive small-group meetings, and computerized decision support or a combination of some of these interventions.[65,67–70] In one study, reminders had the largest average effect and were especially influential for prevention.[68] Some examples of reminders include provider prompts (email and reminder cards); computer assisted treatment plans; and patient prompts (telephone and email reminders). Interventions targeted at specific barriers and combined interventions appear to be more effective.[65,67] More education does not appear to be necessary because clinicians are aware of the available treatments; however, all therapeutic modalities were not consistently used.

A checklist or other reminder system would seem appropriate. As patient-mediated strategies to promote guidelines are also effective, patients with OA could be given a checklist of non-pharmacological treatment options to read in the waiting room. Patients should be encouraged to discuss these options with their doctor. This discussion would serve as a reminder to the physician and stimulate educational and collaborative dialogue between patients and doctors.

GUIDELINE IMPLEMENTATION, QUALITY INDICATORS, AND CONSUMER-DRIVEN HEALTH CARE MODELS

Implementation of clinical guidelines is influenced by several factors, including the performance gap between theory and practice.[65] Upon endorsement of guidelines by the sponsoring body responsible, the process of implementation starts with dissemination of guidelines,[69] encouragement of implementation of guidelines, and the monitoring and evaluation of their impact.[71,72]

In addition to identifying evidence-based implementation strategies, motivation to change requires formal planning and project management processes that need to be explicitly defined a priori. Planning should involve prioritization of recommendations to be implemented, identification of resources that need to be developed, and development of a program evaluation.

This model of implementation integrates project management with the structural systems necessary to support sustained change. A positive predisposition toward continuous quality improvement (CQI) requires leadership that is oriented toward and supports development of CQI policies and processes, such as education and training in CQI, data collection, and management. In addition, a CQI system would integrate these processes with a patient-centered approach to minimizing the risk for adverse events and managing such events as they arise.

SUMMARY

There are numerous evidence-based guidelines available to practicing clinicians that have the potential to improve the quality of health care by promoting interventions of proven benefit and discouraging unnecessary, ineffective, or harmful interventions. Despite the presence of numerous consistent guidelines for OA management and some dissemination attempts, clinical practice does not reflect these recommendations. Future efforts to guide management of OA of the hip or knee are better directed towards implementing practices known to be effective in a context-dependent manner to optimize health care quality.

REFERENCES

1. Lawrence RC, Helmick CG, Arnett FC, et al. Estimates of the prevalence of arthritis and selected musculoskeletal disorders in the United States [see comments]. Arthritis Rheum 1998;41:778–99.
2. Badley E, DesMeules M. Arthritis in Canada: an ongoing challenge. Ottawa: Health Canada; 2003. Cat. # H39-4/14-2003E. ISBN: 0-662-35008-1. Available at: http://www.acreu.ca/pub/aic.html. Accessed March 31, 2010.
3. Glazier RH, Dalby DM, Badley EM, et al. Management of common musculoskeletal problems: a survey of Ontario primary care physicians [see comment]. CMAJ 1998;158:1037–40.
4. Jordan KM, Arden NK, Doherty M, et al. EULAR recommendations 2003: an evidence based approach to the management of knee osteoarthritis: Report of

a Task Force of the Standing Committee for International Clinical Studies Including Therapeutic Trials (ESCISIT) [review]. Ann Rheum Dis 2003;62(12):1145–55.

5. Zhang W, Doherty M, Arden N, et al. EULAR evidence based recommendations for the management of hip osteoarthritis: report of a task force of the EULAR Standing Committee for International Clinical Studies Including Therapeutics (ESCISIT) [comments] [review]. Ann Rheum Dis 2005;64:669–81.

6. Recommendations for the medical management of osteoarthritis of the hip and knee: 2000 update. American College of Rheumatology Subcommittee on Osteoarthritis Guidelines. Arthritis Rheum 2000;43:1905–15.

7. Zhang W, Moskovitz R, Nuki G, et al. OARSI recommendations for the management of hip and knee osteoarthritis, part II: OARSI evidence-based, expert consensus guidelines. Osteoarthritis Cartilage 2008;16:137–62.

8. Hunter D. In the clinic. Osteoarthritis [review]. Ann Intern Med 2007;147. ITC8-1-16.

9. Hunter D, Felson D. Osteoarthritis [review]. BMJ 2006;332:639–42.

10. Centers for Disease Control and Prevention (CDC). Prevalence and impact of chronic joint symptoms–seven states, 1996. MMWR Morb Mortal Wkly Rep 1998;47:345–51.

11. Dunlop DD, Manheim LM, Song J, et al. Arthritis prevalence and activity limitations in older adults. Arthritis Rheum 2001;44:212–21.

12. Centers for Disease Control and Prevention (CDC). Prevalence of disabilities and associated health conditions among adults–United States, 1999 [erratum appears in MMWR Morb Mortal Wkly Rep 2001;50(8):149]. MMWR Morb Mortal Wkly Rep 2001;50:120–5.

13. Guccione AA, Felson DT, Anderson JJ, et al. The effects of specific medical conditions on the functional limitations of elders in the Framingham Study. Am J Public Health 1994;84:351–8.

14. Centers for Disease Control and Prevention (CDC). Arthritis prevalence and activity limitations–United States, 1990. MMWR Morb Mortal Wkly Rep 1994;43: 433–8.

15. Woolf AD, Pfleger B. Burden of major musculoskeletal conditions [review]. Bull World Health Organ 2003;81:646–56.

16. Lopez AD, Murray CC. The global burden of disease, 1990–2020. Nat Med 1998; 4:1241–3.

17. Centers for Disease Control and Prevention (CDC). National and state medical expenditures and lost earnings attributable to arthritis and other rheumatic conditions–United States, 2003. MMWR Morb Mortal Wkly Rep 2007;56:4–7.

18. Misso ML, Pitt VJ, Jones KM, et al. Quality and consistency of clinical practice guidelines for diagnosis and management of osteoarthritis of the hip and knee: a descriptive overview of published guidelines [review]. Med J Aust 2008;189: 394–9.

19. Poitras S, Avouac J, Rossignol M, et al. A critical appraisal of guidelines for the management of knee osteoarthritis using appraisal of guidelines research and evaluation criteria [review]. Arthritis Res Ther 2007;9:R126.

20. Pencharz JN, Grigoriadis E, Jansz GF, et al. A critical appraisal of clinical practice guidelines for the treatment of lower-limb osteoarthritis [review]. Arthritis Res 2002;4:36–44.

21. DeHaan MN, Guzman J, Bayley MT, et al. Knee osteoarthritis clinical practice guidelines – how are we doing? J Rheumatol 2007;34:2099–105.

22. Jawad AS. Analgesics and osteoarthritis: are treatment guidelines reflected in clinical practice? [review]. Am J Ther 2005;12:98–103.

23. Ortiz E. Market withdrawal of Vioxx: is it time to rethink the use of COX-2 inhibitors? J Manag Care Pharm 2004;10:551–4.
24. Felson DT, Lawrence RC, Hochberg MC, et al. Osteoarthritis: new insights. Part 2: treatment approaches [comment] [review]. Ann Intern Med 2000;133:726–37.
25. Wolfe MM, Lichtenstein DR, Singh G. Gastrointestinal toxicity of nonsteroidal antiinflammatory drugs [comment] [review]. N Engl J Med 1999;340:1888–99 [erratum appears in N Engl J Med 1999;341(7):548].
26. Todd PA, Clissold SP. Naproxen. A reappraisal of its pharmacology, and therapeutic use in rheumatic diseases and pain states [review]. Drugs 1990;40: 91–137.
27. Gardiner P, Graham R, Legedza AT, et al. Factors associated with herbal therapy use by adults in the United States. Altern Ther Health Med 2007;13:22–9.
28. Messier SP, Loeser RF, Miller GD, et al. Exercise and dietary weight loss in overweight and obese older adults with knee osteoarthritis: the arthritis, diet, and activity promotion trial [see comment]. Arthritis Rheum 2004;50(5):1501–10.
29. Hutchings A, Calloway M, Choy E, et al. The Longitudinal Examination of Arthritis Pain (LEAP) study: relationships between weekly fluctuations in patient-rated joint pain and other health outcomes. J Rheumatol 2007;34:2291–300.
30. Jordan KM, Sawyer S, Coakley P, et al. The use of conventional and complementary treatments for knee osteoarthritis in the community. Rheumatology 2004;43: 381–4.
31. Ettinger WHJ, Burns R, Messier SP, et al. A randomized trial comparing aerobic exercise and resistance exercise with a health education program in older adults with knee osteoarthritis. The Fitness Arthritis and Seniors Trial (FAST) [see comments]. JAMA 1997;277:25–31.
32. Roddy E, Zhang W, Doherty M, et al. Aerobic walking or strengthening exercise for osteoarthritis of the knee? A systematic review [see comments] [review]. Ann Rheum Dis 2005;64:544–8.
33. Roddy E, Zhang W, Doherty M, et al. Evidence-based recommendations for the role of exercise in the management of osteoarthritis of the hip or knee–the MOVE consensus [see comments] [review]. Rheumatology 2005;44:67–73.
34. Schattner A. Review: both aerobic and home-based quadriceps strengthening exercises reduce pain and disability in knee osteoarthritis. ACP J Club 2005; 143:71.
35. Mancuso CA, Ranawat CS, Esdaile JM, et al. Indications for total hip and total knee arthroplasties. Results of orthopaedic surveys. J Arthroplasty 1996;11: 34–46.
36. Liang MH, Larson MG, Cullen KE, et al. Comparative measurement efficiency and sensitivity of five health status instruments for arthritis research. Arthritis Rheum 1985;28:542–7.
37. Roos E, Nilsdotter A, Toksvig-Larsen S. Patient expectations suggest additional outcomes in total knee replacement [abstract]. Arthritis Rheum 2002;46(Suppl 9): 199.
38. Cohen J. Statistical power analysis for the behavioral sciences. New York: Academic Press; 1977.
39. Katz JN, Mahomed NN, Baron JA, et al. Association of hospital and surgeon procedure volume with patient-centered outcomes of total knee replacement in a population-based cohort of patients age 65 years and older. Arthritis Rheum 2007;56:568–74.
40. Herndon JH, Davidson SM, Apazidis A. Recent socioeconomic trends in orthopaedic practice. J Bone Joint Surg Am 2001;83:1097–105.

41. Winslow CM, Kosecoff JB, Chassin M, et al. The appropriateness of performing coronary artery bypass surgery. JAMA 1988;260:505–9.
42. Moseley JB, O'Malley K, Petersen NJ, et al. A controlled trial of arthroscopic surgery for osteoarthritis of the knee [see comment]. N Engl J Med 2002;347: 81–8 [summary for patients in J Fam Pract 2002;51(10):813].
43. Hall MJ, Lawrence L. Ambulatory surgery in the United States, 1996. Adv Data 1998;(300):1–16.
44. Brinker MR, O'Connor DP, Pierce P, et al. Utilization of orthopaedic services in a capitated population. J Bone Joint Surg Am 2002;84:1926–32.
45. Englund M, Guermazi A, Gale D, et al. Incidental meniscal findings on knee MRI in middle-aged and elderly persons. N Engl J Med 2008;359:1108–15.
46. Bhattacharyya T, Gale D, Dewire P, et al. The clinical importance of meniscal tears demonstrated by magnetic resonance imaging in osteoarthritis of the knee [comment]. J Bone Joint Surg Am 2003;85:4–9.
47. Callahan CM, Drake BG, Heck DA, et al. Patient outcomes following tricompart-mental total knee replacement. A meta-analysis. JAMA 1994;271:1349–57.
48. Ethgen O, Bruyere O, Richy F, et al. Health-related quality of life in total hip and total knee arthroplasty. A qualitative and systematic review of the literature [review]. J Bone Joint Surg Am 2004;86:963–74.
49. Mahomed NN, Barrett J, Katz JN, et al. Epidemiology of total knee replacement in the United States Medicare population. J Bone Joint Surg Am 2005;87:1222–8.
50. Kurtz S, Ong K, Lau E, et al. Projections of primary and revision hip and knee arthroplasty in the United States from 2005 to 2030. J Bone Joint Surg Am 2007;89:780–5.
51. Altman R, Asch E, Bloch D, et al. Development of criteria for the classification and reporting of osteoarthritis. Classification of osteoarthritis of the knee. Diagnostic and therapeutic criteria committee of the American rheumatism association. Arthritis Rheum 1986;29:1039–49.
52. Englund M, Lohmander LS. Risk factors for symptomatic knee osteoarthritis fifteen to twenty-two years after meniscectomy. Arthritis Rheum 2004;50:2811–9.
53. Roos EM, Ostenberg A, Roos H, et al. Long-term outcome of meniscectomy: symptoms, function, and performance tests in patients with or without radio-graphic osteoarthritis compared to matched controls. Osteoarthritis Cartilage 2001;9:316–24.
54. Woolf SH, Grol R, Hutchinson A, et al. Clinical guidelines: potential benefits, limitations, and harms of clinical guidelines [see comment] [review]. BMJ 1999;318: 527–30.
55. Ouwens M, Wollersheim H, Hermens R, et al. Integrated care programmes for chronically ill patients: a review of systematic reviews. Int J Qual Health Care 2005;17:141–6.
56. Chassany O, Boureau F, Liard F, et al. Effects of training on general practitioners' management of pain in osteoarthritis: a randomized multicenter study [see comment]. J Rheumatol 2006;33:1827–34.
57. Pittman MA, Margolin FS. Community health. Crossing the quality chasm: steps you can take. Trustee 2001;54:30–2.
58. IOM (Institute of Medicine). Crossing the Quality Chasm: A New Health System for the 21st Century. Washington, DC: National Academy Press; 2001. Available at: http://www.iom.edu/Global/News%20Announcements/Crossing-the-Quality-Chasm-The-IOM-Health-Care-Quality-Initiative.aspx. Accessed March 31, 2010.
59. Brand C. Translating evidence into practice for people with osteoarthritis of the hip and knee [review]. Clin Rheumatol 2007;26:1411–20.

60. Denoeud L, Mazieres B, Payen-Champenois C, et al. First line treatment of knee osteoarthritis in outpatients in France: adherence to the EULAR 2000 recommendations and factors influencing adherence. Ann Rheum Dis 2005;64:70–4.
61. Mazieres B, Scmidely N, Hauselmann HJ, et al. Level of acceptability of EULAR recommendations for the management of knee osteoarthritis by practitioners in different European countries. Ann Rheum Dis 2005;64:1158–64.
62. Sarzi-Puttini P, Cimmino MA, Scarpa R, et al. Do physicians treat symptomatic osteoarthritis patients properly? Results of the AMICA experience. Semin Arthritis Rheum 2005;35:38–42.
63. Chard J, Dickson J, Tallon D, et al. A comparison of the views of rheumatologists, general practitioners and patients on the treatment of osteoarthritis. Rheumatology 2002;41:1208–10.
64. Rosemann T, Wensing M, Joest K, et al. Problems and needs for improving primary care of osteoarthritis patients: the views of patients, general practitioners and practice nurses. BMC Musculoskelet Disord 2006;7:48.
65. Grol R, Grimshaw J. From best evidence to best practice: effective implementation of change in patients' care [see comment] [review]. Lancet 2003;362:1225–30.
66. Graham ID, Beardall S, Carter AO, et al. The state of the science and art of practice guidelines development, dissemination and evaluation in Canada. J Eval Clin Pract 2003;9:195–202.
67. Grimshaw JM, Shirran L, Thomas R, et al. Changing provider behavior: an overview of systematic reviews of interventions. Med Care 2001;39:II2–45.
68. Grimshaw JM, Eccles MP, Walker AE, et al. Changing physicians' behavior: what works and thoughts on getting more things to work [review]. J Contin Educ Health Prof 2002;22:237–43.
69. Eccles MP, Grimshaw JM. Selecting, presenting and delivering clinical guidelines: are there any "magic bullets". Med J Aust 2004;180:S52–4.
70. Grimshaw J, Eccles M, Thomas R, et al. Toward evidence-based quality improvement. Evidence (and its limitations) of the effectiveness of guideline dissemination and implementation strategies 1966–1998 [review]. J Gen Intern Med 2006;21(Suppl 2):S14–20.
71. Davis DA, Taylor-Vaisey A. Translating guidelines into practice. A systematic review of theoretic concepts, practical experience and research evidence in the adoption of clinical practice guidelines [see comment] [review]. CMAJ 1997;157:408–16.
72. Kresse MR, Kuklinski MA, Cacchione JG. An evidence-based template for implementation of multidisciplinary evidence-based practices in a tertiary hospital setting. Am J Med Qual 2007;22:148–63.

Contextualizing Osteoarthritis Care and the Reasons for the Gap Between Evidence and Practice

Paul Dieppe, BSc, MD, FRCP, FFPH[a], Michael Doherty, MA, MD, FRCP[b],*

KEYWORDS

- Osteoarthritis • Best practice
- National Institute for Clinical Excellence • Contextual care

BEST PRACTICE GUIDELINES FOR THE MANAGEMENT OF OSTEOARTHRITIS

Osteoarthritis (OA) is not an easy condition to manage. It is very heterogeneous, has an unpredictable natural history, and has variable effects on health status. As it primarily affects older adults it is often associated with comorbidities that have significant effects on its impact.[1,2] In addition, there is a wide range of management options available to patients and their health care advisors.[3–5]

Guidelines should help clinicians through this complexity. By synthesizing the best available research evidence on the effectiveness and safety of different interventions, together with expert opinion, they should provide a valuable resource to help advise and treat people with OA. Several authoritative international guidelines on OA management have appeared in recent years,[6] including those from the Osteoarthritis Research Society International[7] and the European League against Rheumatism.[8–10] In addition, individual countries have produced their own guidance, such as that from the United Kingdom's National Institute for Clinical Excellence (NICE)[11] and the American College of Rheumatology[12] (currently undergoing update).

There are many similarities in the advice offered by these different guidelines, suggesting a good deal of consensus on what should and should not be offered to patients with OA.[6] However, several differences also exist, despite the fact that each association has scrutinized the same research evidence base. Some of these differences have been discussed in the literature.[6,13]

[a] Clinical Education Research, Peninsula Medical School, Universities of Exeter and Plymouth, UK
[b] Department Of Rheumatology, Academic Rheumatology, University of Nottingham, Clinical Sciences Building, City Hospital, Nottingham NG5 1PB, UK
* Corresponding author.
E-mail address: Michael.Doherty@nottingham.ac.uk

Clin Geriatr Med 26 (2010) 419–431
doi:10.1016/j.cger.2010.03.004
0749-0690/10/$ – see front matter © 2010 Elsevier Inc. All rights reserved.

Of the various attempts to produce evidence-based recommendations, NICE has perhaps got the closest to evidence-based philosophy.[14] NICE examines all forms of evidence—research, expert opinion, and patient opinion and acceptability—and takes into account economics (cost-effectiveness of interventions) as well as efficacy. For this reason, in addition to the fact that the NICE guidance on the management of OA was published relatively recently and comes to similar conclusions to other contemporary guidance, the authors have chosen to summarize this guideline[11] here, and use it to assess the context within which care is delivered and as the basis for subsequent discussion on the gap between evidence and practice.

THE NICE GUIDELINES ON THE MANAGEMENT OF OSTEOARTHRITIS

There is clear consensus in the literature that empowering self-management alongside help with understanding the condition, encouraging general fitness and moderate activity, keeping muscles strong, and losing weight if obesity is present are the mainstays of the management of OA.[3–5,7,11] Interventions that require medical supervision and/or have potential adverse effects should only be used if these measures are insufficient, and if the patient wants them. Within the NICE guideline these principles are illustrated by a diagram (**Fig. 1**) that shows the simple core measures that everyone with OA should receive at the center of all management. If pain relief is still required then simple safe measures should be tried first (second ring of **Fig. 1**), but there are also treatment options for which there is enough good evidence to warrant possible use in individual patients (outer circle of **Fig. 1**).

It is important that drugs should always be considered as an adjunct to the core management, and are currently only indicated for pain relief. Because NICE gives

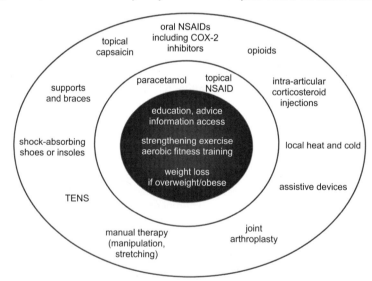

Fig. 1. Summary of NICE recommendations. The inner ring of options should be made available to everyone seeking help for symptomatic osteoarthritis; the next ring includes the 2 therapies that should be first choices for pain management if the innermost ring approaches are insufficient. The outer ring lists all the other interventions that were considered to have enough evidence behind them to be potentially cost effective. This list was based on a review of the evidence that took place in 2007 and 2008. (*Adapted from* National Collaborating Centre for Chronic Conditions. Osteoarthritis: national clinical guideline for care and management in adults. London: Royal College of Physicians, 2008; with permission.)

guidance for practitioners within the budget-limited United Kingdom National Health Service, unlike most other guidelines it includes advice *not to prescribe* certain interventions (eg, intra-articular hyaluronan, acupuncture) for which research evidence is heterogeneous or where there is little or no clear cost-effective benefit. In addition, certain interventions that are recommended in other guidelines, such as glucosamine and chondroitin sulfate, do not appear in the NICE diagram, for reasons discussed below.

CONTEXTUALIZING CARE

NICE strongly emphasizes that management needs to be both individualized and patient-centered.[11] This requires an "holistic" approach with careful patient assessment, taking into account a variety of other variables, including:

1. *OA-related factors* (eg, the site and number of joints involved, the severity of joint damage, and any associated muscle weakness or periarticular problems)
2. *Person-specific factors* (eg, age, sex, ethnicity, socioeconomic and educational status, activity requirements, expectations, and perceptions)
3. *Comorbidity* and concurrent treatments, and the availability, cost, and acceptability of the recommended treatments.

The management of someone with OA, as with any chronic disease, will depend a lot on their individual circumstances. For example, important cultural concerns may have to be addressed: if regular kneeling to pray is a very important part of an individual's life, then it will be more important to them to gain or maintain full flexion of the knee than for a nonreligious individual who lives in a bungalow and spends most of the time in a chair.

Context is discussed further later in this article.

THE GAP BETWEEN EVIDENCE AND PRACTICE

Useful guidelines that exist for the management of people with OA should help health care practitioners deal with the complexity of the condition and their patients. However, there is good evidence that the management of OA remains poor and that most people who seek help for this condition are not managed in accordance with the best practice guidance available.[15–18] Therefore there is, in the management of OA as in so many other chronic diseases, a gap between what evidence-based guidelines recommend and what actually goes on in practice. The remainder of this article discusses this gap.

THE 3 PILLARS OF BEST PRACTICE

One of the reasons for the gap is that recommendations for best practice often focus on just 1 or 2 of the 3 pillars of best practice, which are:

1. Research evidence (including clinical trials)
2. The experienced practitioners' expert opinion and advice
3. The patients' opinion and experience.

All 3 need to have equal weight if we are to claim that we have genuine "best practice" (**Fig. 2**).[14]

As discussed below, guidelines can only do full justice to the research-based evidence.

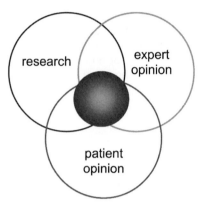

Fig. 2. The three pillars of best practice. Patients will only get the best possible help and advice for them as individuals if the practitioner is able to take account of (1) research evidence (as summarized in guidelines, for example), along with (2) expert opinion, based in part on experience and helping the individualization of therapy through consideration of the contextual factors discussed above, and (3) the patient's opinion, as the individual may have good reason to prefer one therapy to another. (*Data from* Sackett DL, Rosenberg WMC, Gray JAM, et al. Evidence based medicine: what it is and what it isn't. BMJ 1996;312:71–2.)

THE PATHWAY FROM RESEARCH-BASED EVIDENCE TO BEST PRACTICE

There is a complex pathway between the production of the evidence base to the optimum management of the patient, as shown in **Fig. 3**. There are serious problems within each step in the process, contributing to the gap between evidence and practice. Some of these problems are now briefly summarized.

The Production of Evidence Through Trials, Observational Studies, and Other Forms of Research

There are 3 serious problems with the evidence base that we use to develop our guidelines for the treatment of OA:

1. Bias in the evidence available
2. Exclusion of key groups from trials
3. Inappropriate trial methodology.

Bias: The research evidence is hugely biased by vested interests. We do research on interventions that are of interest to, or likely to make money for, a variety of stakeholders in the health care industry. The problem of bias toward pharmaceutical research has been particularly well documented, both in general,[19] and in rheumatology,[20] and is discussed further below.

In addition, the problem of negative publishing bias is well recognized[21]; the vested interest groups, along with journal editors, are much more interested in the positive trial than the negative one. Small trials may provide biased answers that are contradictory to data obtained from larger trials, for a variety of reasons,[22] and several other biases exist within our data.[23]

It is likely that there are a large number of efficacious interventions available and in use for the management of OA that do not appear in any of our guidelines simply because not enough research has been done on them, and published, to provide us with the requisite evidence base.

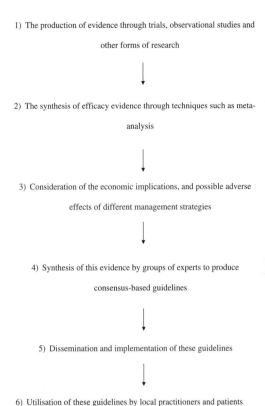

1) The production of evidence through trials, observational studies and
other forms of research

2) The synthesis of efficacy evidence through techniques such as meta-
analysis

3) Consideration of the economic implications, and possible adverse
effects of different management strategies

4) Synthesis of this evidence by groups of experts to produce
consensus-based guidelines

5) Dissemination and implementation of these guidelines

6) Utilisation of these guidelines by local practitioners and patients

Fig 3. The pathway from evidence to practice. This diagram illustrates some of the many steps between the production of primary research-based evidence on interventions and the utilization of an evidence-based guideline by a practitioner.

In the case of OA management the pharmaceutical bias is particularly well illustrated by a study undertaken by Tallon, Chard, and Dieppe some years ago.[23–25] These investigators examined the evidence base for the management of knee OA, and compared findings on which interventions had an evidence base, with the views of patients and practitioners on which interventions they would most like evidence about. There was a big mismatch (**Table 1**). The evidence base was dominated by trials on drugs and observational studies on surgery, nearly all of which favored the intervention being tested, and within which there is good evidence of "sponsorship bias."[25] Patients and practitioners prioritized research on education, physical therapy, and complementary and alternative approaches.[23]

Pharmaceutical industry bias in OA trials is also apparent within the published data on glucosamine.[26,27] Analysis of industry-funded studies of glucosamine sulfate show a moderate effect size (ES 0.47–0.55), compared with virtually no effect (ES 0.05–0.16) in studies that were independent of Industry.[27]

Trial subject selections and exclusions: The generalizability of data from randomized clinical trials and other types of study depends on the patients recruited into the studies. Selection bias is crucially important. Most participants in OA trials are recruited from secondary care and the results of such studies are not readily generalizable to the more common person with OA in the community.[28] Also, the majority of trials focus on knee OA and data derived at one joint site (eg, the knee) may not be

Table 1 Trials of different interventions for knee osteoarthritis up to 1998			
Intervention	Number (%)	% RCTs	% Positive
Drugs	418 (62)	70	95
Surgery	156 (23)	11	91
Physical interventions	35 (5.2)	37	86
Education/Behavioral	29 (4.3)	45	76
Complementary/Alternative (CAM)	37 (5.5)	59	73

The table shows data on published studies of interventions for knee osteoarthritis (1980–1998), showing the numbers published by category of intervention, the percentage of those studies that were randomized clinical trials (RCTs), and the percentage of them that reported a positive outcome in favor of the intervention being investigated. Although nearly all studies were positive, there was still a significant positive association between reporting of sponsorship and a positive finding in favor of the sponsors product (P<.001). These data contrasted with findings from patients with knee osteoarthritis who prioritized education, physical interventions, surgery, and CAM for research.
Data from Refs.[24–26]

generalizable to other sites (eg, the hip or hand).[28] Furthermore, the type of person we are most likely to be treating for OA is often systematically excluded from a trial. For example, as shown by Bartlett and colleagues,[29] older people and people with comorbidities are systematically excluded from the trials of nonsteroidal anti-inflammatory drugs (NSAIDs) in the treatment of OA. And yet it is older people, and people with comorbidities, who dominate those requesting advice and treatment.

Trial design: Most OA clinical trials are based on the standard model of the randomized controlled trial (RCT) in which individuals are randomized to a specific intervention or to a comparator or control group. In reality we never use a single intervention on its own, and in clinical practice we need to take account of all the self-management and other actions being undertaken by our patients to try and help themselves. The classic RCT is only suitable for relatively "simple" interventions, such as a drug that acts as a magic bullet for a specific condition or pathologic process, but there are no "wonder drugs" for OA. Both OA and its management are complex, and we need to adopt the model of complex intervention trials, examining packages of care, the interaction between various components of management and the processes that lead to improvement, and allowing adaptation in response to preferences and treatment responses (adaptive trials) if we are to move our understanding of OA management forward.[30]

These are serious criticisms of the evidence base, applicable to OA and many other chronic conditions, and considered by some to be fatal flaws in the evidence-based movement when it is applied to chronic disease management.[31–33]

The Synthesis of Efficacy Evidence Through Techniques such as Meta-Analysis

Evidence synthesis is only as good as the evidence available (see above). Furthermore, it implies a spurious level of accuracy and certainty within the evidence—with claims, for example, that the effect size for treatment x is 0.35 compared with only 0.25 for treatment y, resulting in the recommendation that we should use x. It is easy to forget that this evidence comes from groups of patients, some of whom will have responded to x and y, and some of whom not, so some patients who are nonresponders to x might do much better with y.

Meta-analyses can also produce different results for the same intervention. As outlined above, small trials are known to produce a bias toward positive results,[22] so some, but by no means all meta-analyses exclude small trials. An example of an area in OA management where the different approaches led to different conclusions is the use of chondroitin sulfate. One meta-analysis that only included trials with a group size of 100 patients or more suggested that this intervention had no efficacy,[34] in contrast to a meta-analysis that included all trials, which concluded that it was efficacious.[35]

Furthermore, there is often marked heterogeneity of RCT results, with some trials being positive and some negative for reasons that are not always clear. For example, the data for glucosamine in OA is very heterogeneous and meta-analyses that include all or most trials report benefit.[36,37] However, separating out the different preparations of glucosamine shows that the hydrochloride is ineffective and that positive results are only observed with the sulfate. Furthermore, as mentioned above, we have to be suspicious that pharmaceutical funding bias is adversely affecting both trials and meta-analyses. Thus, even after vast investment in numerous RCTs, meta-analysis of the combined results may still be inconclusive.

Consideration of the Economic Implications, and Possible Adverse Effects of Different Management Strategies

This is rarely done, partly because it is difficult.

Data on adverse events are not collected in standard ways, and adverse events are most likely to occur in the groups who are routinely excluded from trials (older people and those with comorbidities). RCTs are not sensitive at detecting anything other than very common adverse events, and large observational studies are a better form of evidence to assess safety. So robust data on adverse events often only becomes apparent after widespread adoption of a treatment.

Similarly, economic data are often unavailable, and cannot be included in the consideration of the relative benefits of different approaches to management.

So we do not know about the real risk-benefit ratio or the relative cost benefits of agents such as NSAIDs, commonly used in the management of patients with OA.[38]

Synthesis of This Evidence by Groups of Experts to Produce Consensus-Based Guidelines

Guidelines are produced by committees, therefore the outcome inevitably depends on who sits on them. Committees are usually dominated by doctors, especially hospital-based specialists, and rarely have meaningful input from patients. This fact is likely to mean that our 3 pillars of best-practice development (**Fig. 2**) are not given equal weight.

This is not necessarily due to lack of good intent. Full integration of the views of all key stakeholder groups is difficult to achieve and is expensive, and the resources are often not there to support this.

A further problem is the inevitable gap between the production of evidence, its publication, its subsequent incorporation into meta-analyses (when relevant), and the development of the guideline. Any guideline is likely to be a good 2 years out of date at the time of publication.

Dissemination and Implementation of These Guidelines

Any guideline that is developed is usually *disseminated* widely within the health care profession, but this, of course, does not ensure that it is given any attention. General practitioners in particular are flooded with guidelines and "authoritative information" on how to treat their patients. A guideline on OA is unlikely to appear as exciting or important to them as many of the other things with which they are bombarded.

Guidelines are rarely disseminated to other stakeholders, for example, the patients themselves, their carers, pharmacists, physiotherapists, and other members of the health delivery team.

Implementation of change for the better is very different from dissemination of information. We know that making health-related information available does not, on its own, change behavior. If it did we would have very few problems with obesity or smoking-related disorders. One of the major problems that we have with the management of chronic diseases like OA is that we do not know how to change for the better the behaviors of either the patients or their practitioners.

One approach that we know to be effective in primary care is the use of target-based incentives with financial implications, such as the United Kingdom "QOF" (Quality and Outcomes Framework) system.[39] This system works well when there are accepted goals and readily measured indicators of successful treatment outcome (eg, a defined blood pressure range, a defined level of cholesterol or renal glomerular filtration rate). However, application of such a system to OA is more challenging. Although we might be able to define appropriate targets for management (as outlined by NICE[11]), we need to develop and agree valid and readily measured indicators of good management that can be applied in primary care, such as keeping pain levels below a certain point, or making sure that physical activity is maintained to the level recommended for prevention of cardiovascular disease.

Utilization of Guidelines by Practitioners and Patients

Even if we get to a point where there is good evidence about a management plan that is recommended by a guideline group that disseminates the information well and provides incentives to implementation, individual patients and practitioners may not comply.

Compliance is dependent on individual values and experiences. Many people with OA do not seek medical help, some for very good reasons.[15–18] And even if they do seek help, the professionals they see may not provide the best care. A key barrier to better provision of care for people with OA is negative attitudes, as illustrated by a recent qualitative study by Chard.[40] He found that most GPs and rheumatologists that he interviewed thought that they had very little to offer their patients with OA, unless they needed surgery, and that they found the condition and patients with it "boring." The patients themselves wanted help with self-management, rather than doctor-led interventions, but they too often failed to seek help in the belief that health care professionals had little or nothing to offer them.

One of the reasons for the negativity amongst clinicians may be the fact that OA has a very low priority in undergraduate and postgraduate training.[41] The musculoskeletal curriculum is delivered predominantly by hospital-based specialists whose main interest and emphasis is usually on inflammatory multisystem disorders. Even in rheumatology training OA, the most prevalent arthropathy, is given relatively little attention. An example of the way in which rheumatologists are given a covert message that OA is not very important comes from the position that sections on OA occupy in 2 of the current standard textbooks of rheumatology: in *Rheumatology*[42] OA is in the second of the two volumes, in the 13th of 17 sections, and in the *Oxford Textbook of Rheumatology*[43] it is again in the second volume, in article 15 of 19 chapters on specific conditions. Readers get to know about very rare conditions such as "multicentric reticulohistiocytosis" before they read about OA. Another telling example comes from the update sessions that take place at rheumatology meetings: the inflammatory arthropathies get subdivided into all sorts of aspects and categories, with different sessions on pathogenesis, clinical features, and treatment, while if OA is included at all, someone may be asked to cover everything about it in just one session.

COMORBIDITY AND COMPLEXITY

These aspects of OA were mentioned in the first paragraph of this article, and they represent another major barrier to the implementation of good management in OA, and possible explanation of the gap between evidence and practice.

OA is a disease of older people. It is associated with obesity (and therefore diabetes, hypertension, and other associated disorders), as well as other age-related conditions including cardiovascular disease, reduced renal function, and sensory deficits. Many older people are also socioeconomically disadvantaged, and have psychological distress.

We know that both comorbidities and psychosocial factors have a huge influence on the pain and functional problems of people with OA.[1,2] For example, in a study of disability in older adults with musculoskeletal pain, Ayis and colleagues found that loss of visual acuity was a huge risk factor for the development of severe locomotor disability.[1] We infer form these and other similar data that OA alone is generally not all that disabling, but if one has some other problem as well, such as poor vision that makes one more likely to miss a step or stair, then one can become severely disabled.

As already mentioned, evidence-based guidelines are derived from data collected from people with a single disease—those without comorbidity or complexity.[30] Therefore, evidence-based medicine (EBM) and guidelines do not work well in older people with chronic disease. Work published by Cynthia Boyd and her colleagues a few years ago illustrated this beautifully.[44,45] These investigators showed that older people who come to see their doctors might have several conditions requiring management by best evidence–based guidelines. But attempts to apply the guidelines might lead to conflicting advice. While it might be best to use a thiazide diuretic for the hypertension, for example, this might be contraindicated by the presence of gout complicating osteoarthritis. Similarly, the use of NSAIDs for OA can compromise blood pressure control and corticosteroid injections can temporarily destabilize blood sugar levels in a patient with both OA and diabetes.

So, the art of medicine is as important as the science for good care of older people with chronic diseases like OA.

THE ART OF MEDICINE AND THE CONTEXT OF CARE

The "art of medicine" involves good communication, compassion, and caring. It is about individualizing treatment and finding the person behind the patient, and is centered around the clinical encounter between patient and health care professional.[46,47]

Good communication allows the health care professional to find out what matters most to an individual, and to treat them as a whole person rather than someone with a disease (or set of diseases). As an example, based on data quoted earlier, someone with painful lower limb OA who is having trouble getting about may gain more from good treatment of their visual problems or depression, than from any attempt to treat their pain. *Compassion and caring* work better than most of the other interventions that we use. The authors were recently involved in studies that showed that the context effects (placebo effect) that accompany the interventions used in the management of OA are of more value than the interventions themselves.[48] For example, the standardized mean effect size (ES: where 0.2 is considered small, 0.5 is moderate, and 0.8 is large) for pain relief in RCTs is 0.25 (95% confidence interval [CI] 0.16, 0.34) for nonpharmacologic OA treatments and 0.39 (95% CI 0.31, 0.47) for pharmacologic treatments, whereas the pooled ES for pain relief from placebo (the standardized mean difference between baseline and end point) in OA RCTs is significantly higher at 0.51 (95% CI 0.46–0.55). This ES is even higher at 0.71 (95% CI 0.64, 0.78) in trials with no escape analgesia, perhaps reflecting greater expectation from treatments that do not require such "rescue." The authors have expanded on how and why this might be, and the implications for practice, elsewhere.[49]

The value of a good, caring health care professional can be huge. This might be called an effect of the "microenvironment" or contexts in which we work. The "macro-environment" and contexts matter as well (the example of religious practices was mentioned earlier). The response of people to interventions depend on the meanings that they attach to them, and thus on the culture in which they live.[50,51] So the good management of OA is highly context dependent. Although the "placebo" or meaning response is considered a major nuisance in RCTs, in the context of clinical practice the optimization of contextual and meaning responses, through enhanced care, could greatly benefit people with OA.[49] In audits of medical care, including for OA,[15] common patient complaints are:

- That the doctor was "too busy" to listen or to give time to assess the problem
- That the doctor undertook only a brief examination, or no examination at all
- That the doctor did not appreciate or address key concerns
- That the doctor did not rate the condition as important and underrated the severity of the patient's pain and distress
- That the doctor did not give a return appointment to follow up the outcome.

Conversely, when a practitioner gives a patient their focused and unhurried attention in a confidential environment, listens to them, undertakes a thorough examination and assessment, explains in understandable terms what is happening, addresses concerns, and provides a way forward, the patient experiences a "good deal." This in itself is a treatment that can have a real biologic effect on the patient, alleviating distress and improving pain and function.[49] If we all capitalized fully on optimizing contextual responses, this would be a truly "major treatment advance" in OA.

A WAY FORWARD: CONTEXTUALIZING OSTEOARTHRITIS CARE

OA is common and important—people with it deserve the best available help.

There are two sides to that:

1. The patient: self-management and taking responsibility is as important as anything that the health care professionals can offer.
2. The health care professionals: they need to realize the shortcomings of EBM and guidelines in the management of complexity and comorbidities in older people, and to understand the importance of context, communication, and caring.

This means that we need a different framework and model for the care of older people with chronic disease. The simple biomedical model does not work for people with multiple problems; the biopsychosocial model of disease and illness is more appropriate.[52,53] In addition, the complexity of these persons' problems and the inter-actions of disease and illness issues with their social and cultural backgrounds and position, and health beliefs, means we need a much more flexible, adaptive model of care than that dictated to us by the rigors of EBM guidelines and protocols. One such approach is to use a "toolbox" of options to be discussed between patients and their health care providers.[54] This and other models that embrace true "shared decision making" are more appropriate for the management of people with OA than prescriptive models of care.

With respect to evidence-based guideline development, we also need to: (1) incorporate what we learn from all 3 forms of evidence, and (2) adapt clinical trial designs to make the results more informative and generalizable to people with OA in practice.

REFERENCES

1. Ayis S, Ebrahim S, Williams S, et al. Determinants of reduced walking speed in people with musculoskeletal pain. J Rheumatol 2007;34:1905–12.
2. Kadam UT, Croft PR. Clinical co-morbidity in osteoarthritis: associations with physical function in older patients in family practice. J Rheumatol 2007;34:1899–904.
3. Dieppe PA, Lohmander SL. Pathogenesis and management of pain in osteoarthritis. Lancet 2005;365:965–73.
4. Juni P, Reichenbach S, Dieppe P. Osteoarthritis: rational approach to treating the individual. Best Pract Res Clin Rheumatol 2006;20:721–40.
5. Neame R, Doherty M. Managing osteoarthritis. Practitioner 2003;247:775–9.
6. Zhang W, Moskowitz RW, Nuki G, et al. OARSI recommendations for the management of hip and knee osteoarthritis. Part I: critical appraisal of existing treatment guidelines and systematic review of current research evidence. Osteoarthritis Cartilage 2007;15:981–1000.
7. Zhang W, Moskowitz RW, Nuki G, et al. OARSI recommendations for the management of hip and knee osteoarthritis. Part II: OARSI evidence-based, expert consensus guidelines. Osteoarthritis Cartilage 2008;16:137–62.
8. Jordan KM, Arden N, Doherty M, et al. EULAR Recommendations: an evidence based medicine approach to the management of knee osteoarthritis. Report of a Task Force of the Standing Committee of Clinical Trials and International Studies. Ann Rheum Dis 2003;62:1145–55.
9. Zhang W, Doherty M, Arden N, et al. EULAR recommendations: an evidence based medicine approach to the management of hip osteoarthritis. Report of a Task Force of the Standing Committee of Clinical Trials and International Studies. Ann Rheum Dis 2005;64:669–81.
10. Zhang W, Doherty M, Leeb BF, et al. EULAR evidence-based recommendations for the management of hand osteoarthritis. Report of a Task Force of the EULAR Standing Committee of Clinical Trials and International Studies Including Therapeutics (ESCISIT). Ann Rheum Dis 2007;66:377–88.
11. NICE and Royal College of Physicians Guidelines on Osteoarthritis. Osteoarthritis - national clinical guideline for care and management in adults. 2008. Available at: http://guidance.nice.org.uk/CG59. Accessed March 30, 2010.
12. Altman RD, Hochberg MC, Moskowitz RW, et al. Recommendations for the medical management of osteoarthritis of the hip and knee: 2000 update. Arthritis Rheum 2000;43(9):1905–15.
13. Roddy E, Doherty M. Differences between the ACR and EULAR guidelines on management of knee osteoarthritis. Rheum Dis Clin North Am 2003;29:717–31.
14. Sackett DL, Rosenberg WMC, Gray JAM, et al. Evidence based medicine: what it is and what it isn't. BMJ 1996;312:71–2.
15. OA Nation. 2004. Available at: www.arthritiscare.org.uk/PublicationsandResources/Forhealthprofessionals/OANation. Accessed March 30, 2010.
16. Sanders C, Donovan JL, Dieppe P. Unmet need for joint replacement: a qualitative investigation of barriers to treatment among individuals with severe pain and disability of the hip and knee. Rheumatology 2004;43:353–7.

17. DeHaan MN, Guzman J, Bayley MT, et al. Knee osteoarthritis clinical practice Guidelines. How are we doing? J Rheumatol 2007;34:2099–105.
18. Thorstensson CA, Gooberman-Hill R, Adamson J, et al. Help-seeking behaviour among people living with chronic hip or knee pain in the community. BMC Musculoskelet Disord 2010;10:153.
19. Angell M. The truth about drug companies: how they deceive us and what to do about it. New York: Random House; 2004.
20. Dieppe P. Evidence-based medicine or medicines-based evidence? Ann Rheum Dis 1998;57:385–6.
21. Sterne JA, Gavaghan D, Egger M. Publication and related bias in meta-analysis: power of statistical tests and prevalence in the literature. J Clin Epidemiol 2000; 53:1119–29.
22. Harbord R, Egger M, Sterne J. A modified test for small-study effects in meta-analysis of controlled trials with binary endpoints. Stat Med 2006;25: 3443–57.
23. Tallon D, Chard J, Dieppe P. Exploring the priorities of patients with osteoarthritis of the knee. Arthritis Care Res 2000;13:312–9.
24. Chard J, Tallon D, Dieppe P. Epidemiology of research into interventions for the treatment of osteoarthritis of the knee joint. Ann Rheum Dis 2000;59:414–8.
25. Tallon D, Chard J, Dieppe P. Relation between agendas of the research community and the research consumer. Lancet 2000;355:2037–40.
26. Chard J, Dieppe P. Glucosamine for osteoarthritis: magic, hype, or confusion? BMJ 2001;322:1439–40.
27. Vlad SC, La Valley MP, McAlindon TE, et al. Glucosamine for pain in osteoarthritis. Why do trial results differ? Arthritis Rheum 2007;56:2267–77.
28. Doherty M, Dougados M. Evidence-based management of osteoarthritis: practical issues relating to the data. Best Pract Res Clin Rheumatol 2001;15(4): 517–25 Bailliere.
29. Bartlett C, Doyal L, Ebrahim S, et al. The causes and effects of socio-demographic exclusions from clinical trails. Health Technol Assess 2005;38:1–152.
30. Craig P, Dieppe P, Macintyre S, et al. Developing and evaluating complex interventions: the new MRC guidance. BMJ 2008;337:1665.
31. Charlton B, Miles A. The rise and fall of EBM. QJM 1998;91:371–4.
32. Christiansen C, Lou JQ. Ethical considerations related to evidence-based practice. Am J Occup Ther 2001;55:345–9.
33. Dieppe P, Szebenyi B. Evidence based rheumatology. J Rheumatol 2000;27:4–7.
34. Reichenbach S, Sterchi R, Scherer M, et al. Meta-analysis: chondroitin for osteoarthritis of the knee or hip. Ann Intern Med 2007;146:580–90.
35. McAlindon TE, LaValley MP, Gulin JP, et al. Glucosamine and chondroitin for treatment of osteoarthritis: a systematic quality assessment and meta-analysis. JAMA 2000;283:1469–75.
36. Towheed TE, Maxwell L, Anastassiades TP, et al. Glucosamine therapy for treating osteoarthritis. The Cochrane Library 2005;2:CD002946.
37. Richy F, Bruyere O, Ethgen O, et al. Structural and symptomatic efficacy of glucosamine and chondroitin in knee osteoarthritis: a comprehensive meta-analysis. Arch Intern Med 2003;163:1514–22.
38. Dieppe P, Bartlett C, Davey P, et al. Balancing benefits and harms: the example of non-steroidal anti-inflammatory drugs. BMJ 2004;329:458–9.
39. 'QOF' (Quailty and Outcomes Framework) system. Department of Health, 2004 (updated 2009). Available at: www.dh.gov.uk/en/Healthcare/Primarycare/ Primarycarecontracting/QOF. Accessed March 30, 2010.

40. Chard J. Investigation of services for osteoarthritis. PhD Thesis, University of Bristol, 2005.
41. Woolf AD, Walsh NE, Akesson K. Global core recommendations for a musculo-skeletal undergraduate curriculum. Ann Rheum Dis 2004;63:517–24.
42. Hochberg MC, Silman AJ, Smolen JS, et al, editors. Rheumatology. 4th edition. London (UK): Mosby Elsevier; 2008.
43. Oxford Textbook of Rheumatology. Maddison PJ, Woo P, Isenberg D, et al, editors. Oxford: Oxford University Press; 2004.
44. Boyd CM, Darer J, Boult C, et al. Clinical practice guidelines and quality of care for older patients with multiple comorbid disease. JAMA 2005;294:716–24.
45. Boyd C, Ritchie C, Tipton E, et al. From bedside to bench: summary from the American Geriatrics Society/National Institute on Aging Research Conference on Co-morbidity and Multiple Morbidity in Older Adults. Aging Clin Exp Res 2008;20:181–8.
46. Goodrich J, Cornwell J. Seeing the person in the patient. London: King's Fund; 2008.
47. Dieppe P, Rafferty A, Kitson A. The clinical encounter—the focal point of patient-centred care. Health Expect 2002;5:279–81.
48. Zhang W, Robertson J, Jones A, et al. The placebo response and its determi-nants in osteoarthritis—meta-analysis of randomised controlled trials. Ann Rheum Dis 2008;67:1716–23.
49. Doherty M, Dieppe PA. The "placebo" response in osteoarthritis and its implica-tions for clinical practice. Osteoarthritis Cartilage 2009;17:1255–62.
50. Moerman DE, Jonas WB. Deconstructing the placebo effect and finding the meaning response. Ann Intern Med 2002;136:471–6.
51. Kleinman A. The illness narratives: suffering, healing and the human condition. London: Basic Books (Harper Collins); 1988.
52. Engel GL. The need for a new medical model: a challenge for biomedicine. Science 1977;196:129–36.
53. Jordan KM, Sawyer S, Coakley P, et al. The use of conventional and complementary treatments for knee osteoarthritis in the community. Rheumatology 2004;43:381–4.
54. Dieppe P. From protocols to principles, from guidelines to toolboxes: aids to the good management of osteoarthritis. Rheumatology 2001;40:841–2.

Transforming Osteoarthritis Care in an Era of Health Care Reform

William H. Gruber, PhD[a],*, David J. Hunter, MBBS, PhD, FRACP[b,c]

KEYWORDS

- Osteoarthritis • Elderly • Conservative care • Health reform
- Medical leadership • Broken health care system

"If we don't get health care done now, then no one's health insurance is going to be secure. You're going to continue to see premiums going up at astronomical rates, out of pocket costs going up at astronomical rates, and people who lose their jobs... finding themselves in a situation where they cannot get health care...* That is not a future I accept for the United States of America."
                                            —*President Barack Obama, July 17, 2009[1]*

The combined national crises of high unemployment (10% at the end of 2009)[2] and giant federal debt (forecasted to reach $18.6 trillion in 2020 or 77% of the gross domestic product [GDP])[3,4] are juxtaposed with a crunch of unsustainable rapid inflation in health costs, a result of a defective preindustrial delivery and payment system that fails in delivery of quality and cost-effective care for patients with chronic illness,[5,6] which is pervasive and costly among the vast majority of the elderly.[7,8] Within a context of urgent national crisis, President Obama and Congress have worked for more than a year on health reform, but legislation[9] is unlikely to contribute significantly to overall cost reduction and improved quality.[10] Given the national economic crises and the likely failure of federal legislation to adequately address the quality and cost challenges, there is a major imperative for physician and hospital leadership to transform the delivery of health care. As the authors describe, the delivery of osteoarthritis (OA) conservative care is now seriously defective,[11,12] but remarkable improvement is now attainable. This forecast is based on leading integrated delivery system (IDS) exemplars making progress in the last decade[13] toward

[a] 3402 Main Campus Drive, Lexington, MA 02421, USA
[b] Department of Rheumatology, Northern Clinical School, University of Sydney, 2065, Sydney, Australia
[c] Division of Research, New England Baptist Hospital, 125 Parker Hill Avenue, Boston, MA 02120, USA
* Corresponding author.
E-mail address: whgruber@comcast.net

Clin Geriatr Med 26 (2010) 433–444
doi:10.1016/j.cger.2010.03.005
0749-0690/10/$ – see front matter © 2010 Elsevier Inc. All rights reserved.

a future best practice delivery of conservative OA care. To provide significant improvement in the quality of care and cost effectiveness for the elderly and frail population with chronic OA and frequently associated comorbidities, the authors recommend the use of innovations tested by a small number of visible key leaders in health care improvement.

A PATIENT PERSPECTIVE: DELIVERY OF OSTEOARTHRITIS CARE

One of the authors is an elder (aged more than 65 years and on Medicare) suffering from OA and multiple comorbidities, common among the 27 million[7] individuals afflicted, of whom a large percentage are elderly.[14] This author's OA and related comorbidities are detrimental to his mobility for desired activities, including walking and golf, and reducing fatigue and pain. The overall provider-patient relationship lacks monitoring of patient-specific outcomes.[15] For a condition that is degenerative and incurable, a strong patient-physician shared vision is critical in the management of OA.[16] This relationship is also crucial for the ability of patients to reach personal goals dependent on age and metrics, including range of motion, ability to stand without pain, and strength of quadriceps.[15,17] Conventional wisdom holds the assumption that an informed patient is able to assume an important role in the management of an illness.[18] This conventional wisdom has been seriously tested by one of the author's efforts to learn about function and pain management options, such as braces,[19] for OA of the knee and the related musculoskeletal condition, spondylolisthesis of the lower back and neck. The complexity of the patient perspective can be seen from the context of a patient surrounded by autonomous caregivers with little communication from provider to provider (**Fig. 1**).[20,21]

In an effort to standardize best care delivery practices, the Osteoarthritis Research Society International (OARSI) has published guidelines for OA conservative care,[22] but currently insurance does not cover a large number of these guidelines and those that are covered allow patients only a predetermined number of visits with preventative services after injury, such as physical therapy.[23,24] The medical profession is consequently not organized to deliver the care needed for patients with OA,[11] as advocated by the OARSI guidelines.

When recommended guidelines are not provided in an integrated delivery system of OA care patients are left in a state of uncertainty and as a consequence suffer potential

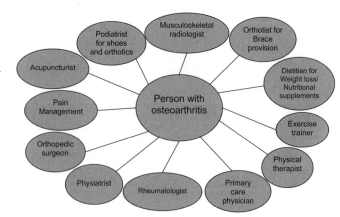

Fig. 1. Now silo-based/lack of evidence-based care in a complex patient situational condition: musculoskeletal/OA case report.

harm to health and decreased quality of life.[25] The impact of comorbid conditions, such as obesity and diabetes, can be seen as a matrix of interaction effects (**Fig. 2**). Obesity is a common comorbid condition among those with OA and total knee and hip replacements,[26] and as noted by Cicuttiniand and colleagues,[27] each kilogram of excess weight increases the risk for OA by 9% to13%. Patients in increasing pain become less active,[28] limiting daily exercise that, if not properly managed, can lead to additional weight gain adding further to joint loading.[29] This comorbid matrix illustrates that without a comprehensive model, patients only receive silo-based care[25] that is focused on one condition, thereby increasing the negative effects of all the comorbidities.

From the patient perspective, what has the medical profession done to assure compliance with recommended guidelines for appropriate patient self-management actions, such as strengthening quadriceps muscles? The conventional wisdom that patients will comply with recommended guidelines if they are given the self-management information and even tools,[18] such as a personal health record, is questionable given that patients are not *integrated* into a systematic feedback loop of information[30] that monitors patients on a regular basis and provides feedback to patients and their providers. Given this reality, the following questions arise: What on-going metrics of patient outcomes does the medical profession maintain? What research has the medical profession carried out to develop improved competence for the key metric guidelines? How many primary care physicians, rheumatologists, or surgeons who care for patients with OA maintain this kind of support and competence for the OARSI evidence-based guidelines on the value of exercise?

From this particular patient's perspective, some examples of the OARSI guidelines that are challenging to implement in the traditional health care setting are: (1) aerobic and strengthening exercise; (2) braces; (3) injections, such as Synvisc (Genzyme Corp, Cambridge, MA, USA); (4) shoe wedges; and (5) personal health record[22] with longitudinal metrics for OA status, such as pain, quadriceps strength, and range of motion. Typically these interventions are delivered by a variety of different health professionals

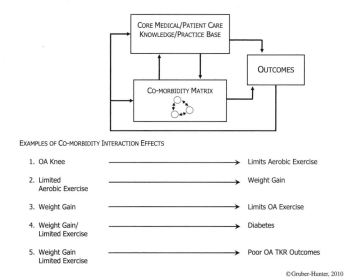

Fig. 2. OA comorbidity negative feedback consequences. *Courtesy of* W. H. Gruber, PhD, Lexington MA; and D. J. Hunter, PhD, Boston, MA.

acting in a silo from the patients' other providers.[21] Patients needs require a strong enabler who coordinates their care,[31] such as exercise, for example, because it can be tedious, time consuming, and even painful. The current lack of transformation practices as applied in this OA case study makes it unlikely that there is patient proactive monitoring for compliance and patient monitoring for the outcomes from exercise.[32] Tracking the longitudinal metrics associated with OA, such as atrophy of the quadriceps, is critical to patients' success.[33] This patient-perspective case study also illustrates the failure of the medical profession to learn from patient observations[34] and thereby test and validate the evidence-based guidelines that are now too sparsely tested[32] given the complexity of the medical problems faced by patients.

OSTEOARTHRITIS PAIN LIFE CYCLE

Patients frequently endure more than a decade in the OA pain life cycle stages (**Fig. 3**). The Robert Wood Johnson Foundation (RWJF) has taken a giant leap in advocating for patient perspective through the collection of what they call observations of daily living (ODL). ODL is a term the RWJF uses to describe "pattern of everyday living,"[34] which can be recorded, gathered, interpreted, and then integrated in the delivery practice models and processes used by the physicians. These ODLs can include range of motion, length of time patients can walk without pain, or sleep disruption caused by pain.

Experts from OARSI have identified an OA pain and loss of functionality life cycle,[22] which is represented in their 25 evidence-based guidelines for the care of OA. As a chronic illness, OA has a pain and loss of functionality cycle that can last for more than a decade, lessening the quality of life until, as the stages go from 0 to III (see **Fig. 3**), patients present to a surgeon with a statement, such as "you reach a point where you know it is time to do something,"[35] wherein there is a move from what should have been conservative care in stages 0 to III into major surgery in stage IV. The OARSI guidelines recommend conservative care in stages 0 to III to limit the use of this highly invasive surgery in stage IV. Although improvements have been made in surgical practice, joint replacement surgery is associated with attendant risk, including infection[36]; is not suitable for many individuals with concomitant morbidities;

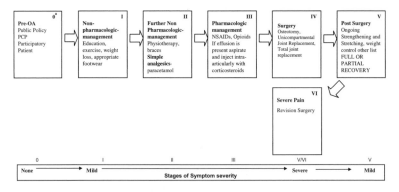

*Stages 0-VI in OA Severity: Zang, et al (2008) OARSI recommendations for the management of hip and knee osteoarthritis, Part II: OARSI evidence-based, expert consensus Guidelines. *Osteoarthritis and Cartilage* 16, 137e162

Fig. 3. Hunter-Gruber OA severity continuum value chain/total life cycle in a population with osteoarthritis. NSAIDs, nonsteroidal antiinflammatory drugs; PCP, primary care physician. *From* Hunter D, Felson D. Osteoarthritis. BMJ 2006;332(7542);641; with permission.

and requires months of rehabilitation for recovery. After recovery, patients should go into stage V, which is prolonged protection of the knee or hip joint that was made functional with the implant. It has been said that strong quadriceps are the best brace for a knee weakened by OA.[37] Exercise and strengthening, during the pre-surgery stages of OA (see **Fig. 3**), are sustaining forces that drastically increase the success of the total knee replacement (TKR),[38] lower pain, and enable on-going quality-of-life functions,[22] and therefore should be enabled by a health coach integrated into the OA pain cycle. Significant progress has also been achieved in other IDS, such as Partners Healthcare and CareGroup who have set a standard (eg, the recently instituted elder care program at Massachusetts General Hospital) that works to decrease the number of emergency room visits and hospital stays experienced, with a focus on the frail elderly.[39]

MAGNITUDE OF OSTEOARTHRITIS IN THE UNITED STATES

In this era of the health care reform crisis, the case the authors make for OA is timely because the national conversation has closely focused on the burden of cost on the government, insurance companies, employers, and the public. One area of health care that has garnered much attention in the reform debate is chronic illness. This attention is because 75% of the total health expenditures[40] is attributed to the cost of chronic illness, including such comorbid conditions as diabetes, obesity, and hypertension (**Table 1**).[41] People with five or more chronic diseases, typically those aged more than 65 years, make up 68% of total Medicare spending.[42]

Inflation in the cost of health care[43] for patients with OA is likely to continue exceeding the rate of growth in GDP, gaining an ever greater share,[44] and may even exceed the surgical capacity of the medical profession. Resources for the forecasted increase in the numbers of annual total knee and total hip replacements are projected to increase from 600,000 in 2008 to 4 million procedures by 2030.[45] The total cost of this OA epidemic includes more than the direct medical costs associated with treatment because of the significant indirect costs, such as lost productivity[46] and the harm caused to patients with additional comorbidities who have limited coping capability because of the functional limitations and pain caused by OA.[28,47] Thus, the full

Table 1
Personal health spending by diagnostic category and medical condition, selected years 1996 to 2005

Category/Condition[a]	Spending by Year (Billions of Dollars)		Share of 2005 Spending (%)
	1996	2005	
Circulatory System	150.9	253.9	17
Heart conditions	81.0	123.1	8
Cerebrovascular disease	22.9	26.8	2
Hypertension	22.6	50.2	3
Hyperlipidemia	4.6	22.8	2
Musculoskeletal	57.9	121.8	8
Osteoarthritis	23.5	48.0	3
Back problems	17.9	40.1	3
Mental Disorders	81.5	142.2	9
Anxiety and depression	30.45	63.2	4

[a] Medical conditions are not all-inclusive, so spending by condition sums to less than category totals.

Data from Roehrig C, Miller G, Lake C, et al. National Health Spending By Medical Condition, 1996–2005. Health Affairs 2009;28(2):w361. Available at: http://content.healthaffairs.org/cgi/content/abstract/28/2/w358. Accessed February 3, 2010.

cost of OA should be seen relative to the cost of comorbid chronic illnesses, such as those summarized in **Table 1**.

As one of the most pervasive chronic illnesses in the United States,[48] OA is expected to increase in number of patients afflicted and cost of care at a high rate over the next several decades because of an increase in the aging population and prevalence of obesity.[49] The 27 million individuals with OA[7] are largely left to self manage a complex chronic illness with little comprehensive guidance or support from the medical profession.[12] In a 2006 study conducted by the Osteoarthritis Initiative,[50] it was estimated that by 2030 approximately 70 million people older than 65 years of age will be at risk for osteoarthritis. This increase will compound the already substantial burden ($128 billion)[40] of cost related to arthritis care and corresponding comorbid conditions[41] (see **Table 1**) on the United States.

FISCAL HEALTH CRISIS: COST OF CHRONIC CARE

The health care system in the United States has for some time been degrading rapidly into an unaffordable crisis of subpar care that at the same time adds to federal deficits reaching unsustainable levels. The Obama administration's budget for fiscal year 2011[4] is estimated at $3.83 trillion and with a deficit of $1.2 trillion for 2011 alone.[51] Deficits and debt have been increasing dramatically; federal debt increased from $5.8 trillion in 2001[52] to approximately $12.7 trillion at the beginning of 2009[52] and is projected to reach more than $18 trillion by 2020.[3,53] A large part of this increase is caused by the estimated increase in total health expenditures, which in 2009 reached $2.6 trillion and are projected to reach $4.7 trillion, or 21.3% of the GDP, by 2019.[54] The largest part of the expense is caused by the total Medicare and Medicaid expenditures estimated to increase from $726 billion in 2010 to an estimated $1.4 trillion in 2020, a decade of federal spending of $10.5 trillion.[4] The Centers for Medicare and Medicaid Services estimates total exhaustion of the Medicare Trust Fund during 2017.[55] Net interest on total federal debt is predicted to increase from $188 billion in 2010 to $840 billion in 2020,[4] effectively quadrupling in size in just 10 years. This giant increase in national health expenditure is caused in part by an increase in the older population, technological advancement, and ineffective delivery/payment system.

HEALTH CARE REFORM IN AN AGE OF NATIONAL CRISES

Dr Jeffrey Flier,[10] dean of Harvard Medical School, strongly articulated a negative view of health care reform for which he gave a failing grade. Dean Flier and other opinion leaders have noted the importance of physicians to take a more proactive role as a stakeholder and participant in the process of health care reform in contrast to the unlikely input of legislation to improve the broken health care system.[56] For a transformation to occur, all stakeholders, including providers and particularly the medical leadership, must take responsibility for motivating and integrating transformational delivery practices into organizational competence.[57]

Dr Donald Berwick, arguably the single most important person in the health care improvement movement and President of the Institute for Healthcare Improvement, is now advocating reform with a focus on population management[58] in the delivery of health care. This shift from the fee-for-service model to population health in the delivery of health care is a new standard for health providers.[21] Population health management falls under Dr Berwick and colleagues'[59] larger quality improvement effort: the "pursuit of three aims: improving the experience of care, improving the health of populations, and reducing per capita costs of health care." Historically, providers did not take responsibility for the health of the population that they served but instead provided care on an episodic basis once a patient became ill.[42] It is a massive rethink in values and practices for providers to set goals for the quality of health care and the cost in delivery to a population of patients.

HEALTH CARE: A PREINDUSTRIAL INDUSTRY

In the current turmoil of competing health care reform advocacy, there has been seriously inadequate attention given to the challenge of the transformation of health care into a new paradigm of future best practice[60] from the existing preindustrial delivery model that lacks organizational oversight in the quality and cost effectiveness of health care. The *New England Journal of Medicine* article "Cottage Industry to Postindustrial Care — The Revolution in Health Care Delivery" by leading experts, including Stephen J. Swensen,[61] Donald Berwick, Brent James, Gary S. Kaplan, and Mark Chassin, documented that health care in the United States is preindustrial[61] with serious, unaffordable cost inflation and variable quality outcomes as compared with industrial sectors of the economy.[61]

TOWARDS INDUSTRIAL HEALTH CARE

The innovations required to bring health care from preindustrial to industrial competence include (projecting ahead 20 to 30 years)

1. Integrated delivery system: a network of organizations linked with providers, such as primary care, specialty groups, and surgical centers[30]
2. Delivery value chain: "disaggregates"[62] the organization into activities that positions the organization so that it can gain the most knowledge of the activity-to-cost relationship
3. Patient-centered medical home (PCMH)[63,64]
4. Research and development for improvement in the delivery of quality, cost effectiveness, and comparative evaluation of medical interventions in patient care[58]
5. Transparency of quality and loss by illness, provided in the IDS[65]
6. Integrated health information technology[66,67]
7. Bundling of fees by outcome for a given medical problem.[68,69]

In the new paradigm delivery model of the PCMH there is a coach integrator of patient care, integrated health information system, metrics, communication among multiple providers, inclusion of comorbidity issues, and connectivity with sensing devices,[66] which are all now largely missing in medical practice for conservative care of OA. This new paradigm can largely be enabled by technology. The exemplars frequently cited are Mayo Clinic, Cleveland Clinic, Kaiser Permanente, Intermountain Healthcare, and Geisinger.[58] Geisinger, for example has started on the path toward an exemplary standard care with their "Proven Care Model."[70]

SUMMARY: OPPORTUNITY FOR EXEMPLARS

The new paradigm of industrial strength, conservative OA care has benefits for multiple stakeholders who can learn from a decade of exemplar medical leadership that has achieved impressive early-stage competence in solutions for comprehensive care of chronic illnesses. This new paradigm is especially important for the elder population, expected to increase by 78 million over 17 years,[71] of which more than half are estimated to show signs of OA[72] at 65 years of age and older and are at an increased risk for other comorbid chronic conditions, which make up 75% of total health expenditures.[40] Given the magnitude of OA costs and the related impact on other chronic comorbidities, a cost savings of 10% to 20%[73,74] would make an extraordinary reduction in the rate of debt incurred by the government from health expenditures.[75] This reduction would foster economic growth, increase personal financial stability, and decrease the burden on caregivers of elderly individuals who are chronically ill.

Medical-leadership collaboration with other stakeholders, such as health insurance companies and employers, is critical for profound improvement in the quality and affordability of health care. Given that these objectives can only be achieved with full participation of medical leadership and the very financial insolvency of the government is in question, an increasing elder population in need of a greater amount of care and a dysfunctional medical system unprepared to deal with this increase provides a strong incentive for progress as targeted in this article.

REFERENCES

1. Brown CB. Obama: don't bet against me. Politico 2009; Available at: http://www.politico.com/news/stories/0709/25091.html. Accessed February 15, 2010.
2. Employment situation summary. Bureau of Labor Statistics. U.S Department of Labor; 2010. Available at: http://www.bls.gov/news.release/empsit.nr0.htm. Accessed February 15, 2010.
3. Weisman J. Wealthy face tax increase: budget projects rising debt despite spending cuts; GOP decries deficits. Wall St J 2010. Available at: http://online.wsj.com/article/SB10001424052748704107204575038733246595218.html. Accessed February 15, 2010.
4. Budget of the U.S. Government FY 2011. Office of Management and Budget; 2010. 178, 146. Available at: http://www.whitehouse.gov/omb/budget/fy2011/assets/budget.pdf. Accessed February 15, 2010.
5. Institute of Medicine. Crossing the quality chasm: a new health system for the 21st century. Washington, DC: National Academy Press; 2001.
6. Hoffman C, Rice DP. Chronic care in America: a 21st century challenge. San Francisco (CA): The Institute for Health and Aging, University of California; 1996.
7. Helmick C, Felson D, Lawrence R, et al. Estimates of the prevalence of arthritis and other rheumatic conditions in the United States. Arthritis Rheum 2008; 58(1):15–25.
8. Yelin E, Murphy L, Cisternas M, et al. Estimates of the prevalence of arthritis and other rheumatic conditions in the United States in 2003, and comparisons to 1997. Arthritis Rheum 2007;56(5):1397–407.
9. Henry E. Obama's first year: strong foundation or house of cards? Available at: http://www.cnn.com/2010/POLITICS/01/20/obama.first.year/index.html. Accessed February 15, 2010.
10. Flier JS. Health 'reform' gets a failing grade. Wall St J 2009. Available at: http://online.wsj.com/article/SB10001424052748704431804574539581994054014.html. Accessed January 29, 2010.
11. Pencharz JN, Grigoriadis E, Jansz GF, et al. A critical appraisal of clinical practice guidelines for the treatment of lower-limb osteoarthritis. Arthritis Res 2002;4:36–44.
12. DeHaan MN, Guzman J, Bayley MT, et al. Knee osteoarthritis clinical practice guidelines – how are we doing? J Rheumatol 2007;34:2099–105.
13. Porter M, Teisberg EE. Redefining healthcare: creating value-based competition on results. Boston: Harvard Business School; 2006.
14. Lawrence RC, Felson DT, Helmick CG, et al. Estimates of the prevalence of arthritis and other rheumatic conditions in the United States. Part II. Arthritis Rheum 2008;58:26–35.

15. McKenzie S, Bridges-Webb C. Doctor-patient treatment goals in the management of osteoarthritis in general practice. Aust Fam Physician 2004;33(11): 959–60.

16. Maly MR, Krupa T. Personal experience of living with knee osteoarthritis among older adults. Disabil Rehabil 2007;29(18):1423–33.

17. Marshall LL, Miller SW. Osteoarthritis in the geriatric patient. J Geriatr Drug Therapy 2000;12(4):21–43. Available at: http://www.informaworld.com/smpp/content~content=a904564096~db=all~jumptype=rss. Accessed March 30, 2010.

18. Bishop G, Brodkey AC. Personal responsibility and physician responsibility — West Virginia's Medicaid plan. N Engl J Med 2006;355(8):756–8.

19. How do braces work. Arthritis Foundation; 2009. Available at: http://www.arthritis.org/how-braces-work.php. Accessed February 3, 2010.

20. Berwick D. Escape from fire: designs for the future of health care. San Francisco (CA): Jossey-Bass; 2004.

21. Shih A, Davis K, Schoenbaum S, et al. Organizing the U.S. health care delivery system for high performance. Commonwealth Fund Report 2008; 98.

22. Zhang W, Moskowitz R, Nuki G, et al. OARSI recommendations for the management of hip and knee osteoarthritis. Part II: OARSI evidence-based, expert consensus guidelines. Osteoarthritis Cartilage 2008;12(2):137–62.

23. Health and Human Services. Covered services - physical therapy. Commonwealth of Massachusetts; 2010. Available at: http://www.mass.gov/?pageID=eohhs2terminal&L=4&L0=Home&L1=Consumer&L2=Insurance+(including+MassHealth)&L3=MassHealth+Information+for+Members&sid=Eeohhs2&b=terminalcontent&f=masshealth_consumer_member_covered_services&csid=Eeohhs2#thera. Accessed February 15, 2010.

24. Insured but not covered. Consumers Union of U.S., Inc. Consumer Reports 2007. Available at: http://www.consumerreports.org/health/insurance/health-insurance-9-07/insured-but-not-covered/0709_health_adjust.htm. Accessed February 15, 2010.

25. Wagner EH, Austin BT, Davis C, et al. Improving chronic illness care: translating evidence into action. Health Aff 2001;20(6):64–78.

26. Grotle M, Hagen KB, Natvig B, et al. Obesity and osteoarthritis in knee, hip and/or hand: an epidemiological study in the general population with 10 years follow-up. BMC Musculoskelet Disord 2008;2(9):132.

27. Cicuttini FM, Baker JR, Spector TD. The association of obesity with osteoarthritis of the hand and knee in women: a twin study. J Rheumatol 1996;7:1221–6.

28. Kudum UT, Croft PR. Clinical comorbidity in osteoarthritis: associations with physical function in older patients in family practice. J Rhematol 2007;34(9):1899–904.

29. Griffin TM, Guilak F. The role of mechanical loading in the onset and progression of osteoarthritis. Exerc Sport Sci Rev 2005;33(4):195–200.

30. Porter ME. A strategy for health care reform — toward a value-based system. N Engl J Med 2009;361(2):109–12.

31. Adleman AM, Graybill M. Integrating a health coach into primary care: reflections from the penn state ambulatory research network. Ann Fam Med 2005;3(Suppl 2):S33–5. DOI: 10.1370/afm.317.

32. Poitras S, Avouac J, Rossignol M, et al. A critical appraisal of guidelines for the management of knee osteoarthritis using appraisal of guidelines research and evaluation criteria. Arthritis Res Ther 2007;9:R126.

33. Burstein D. Tracking longitudinal changes in knee degeneration and repair. J Bone Joint Surg Am 2009;91:51–3.

34. Project Health Design. Rethinking the power and potential of personal health records. 2009 call for proposals-round 2. Robert Wood Johnson Foundation; 2009.
35. Back on the treadmill with a new knee: computerized navigation aids precision during surgery. Healthworks Magazine; 2009. Available at: http://www.emersonhospital.org/about/news/healthworks/documents/HW_winter_09.pdf. Accessed February 15, 2010.
36. Wilson MG, Kelly K, Thornhill TS. Infection as a complication of total knee-replacement arthroplasty. Risk factors and treatment in sixty-seven cases. J Bone Joint Surg Am 1990;72(6):878–83.
37. Shreyasee A, Baker K, Niu J, et al. Quadriceps strength and the risk of cartilage loss and symptom progression in knee osteoarthritis. Arthritis Rheum 2009;60(1): 189–98.
38. Deshmukh R, Hayes J, Pinder I. Does body weight influence outcome after total knee arthroplasty? A 1-year analysis. J Arthroplasty 2002;17(3):315–9.
39. Kowalczyk L. Hospital strains to cut elder care costs: mass. General's effort reflects a national challenge. The Boston Sunday Globe 2009. A19. Available at: http://www.boston.com/news/health/articles/2009/05/17/hospital_strains_to_cut_elder_care_costs/. Accessed February 15, 2010.
40. Chronic disease overview. Centers for Disease Control and Prevention; 2008. Available at: http://www.cdc.gov/NCCdphp/overview.htm#2. Accessed February 15, 2010.
41. Roehrig C, Miller G, Lake C, et al. National health spending by medical condition, 1996–2005. Health Aff 2009;28(2):w361. Available at: http://content.healthaffairs.org/cgi/content/abstract/28/2/w358. Accessed February 15, 2010.
42. Carapenter S. Treating an illness is one thing. What about a patient with many? New York Times 2009. Available at: http://www.nytimes.com/2009/03/31/health/31sick.html. Accessed February 15, 2010.
43. Updated and extended national health expenditure projections 2010–2019. Centers for Medicare and Medicaid Services; 2009. Available at: http://www.cms.hhs.gov/NationalHealthExpendData/downloads/NHE_Extended_Projections.pdf. Accessed January 29, 2010.
44. Maetzel A. The challenges of estimating the National costs of osteoarthritis: are we making progress? J Rheumatol 2002;29:9.
45. Paxton EW, Inacio M, Slipchenko T, et al. The Kaiser Permanente national total joint replacement registry. The Permanente Journal 2008;12(3):12–6. Available at: http://xnet.kp.org/permanentejournal/sum08/joint-replacement.pdf. Accessed February 15, 2010.
46. Centers for Disease Control and Prevention. National and state medical expenditures and lost earnings attributable to arthritis and other rheumatic conditions-United States, 2003. MMWR Morb Mortal Wkly Rep 2007;56:4–7.
47. Powell A, Teichtahl AJ, Wluka AE, et al. Obesity: a preventable risk factor for large joint osteoarthritis which may act through biomechanical factors. Br J Sports Med 2005;39:4–5.
48. Agency for Healthcare Research and Quality. Managing osteoarthritis helping the elderly maintain function and mobility. Research in Action; 2002. Available at: http://www.ahrq.gov/research/osteoria/osteoria.pdf. Accessed March 30, 2010.
49. Analysis of the President's Budgetary proposals for fiscal year 2010. Congressional Budget Office; 2009. Available at: http://www.cbo.gov/ftpdocs/102xx/doc10296/06-16-AnalysisPresBudget_forWeb.pdf. Accessed February 15, 2010.

50. Osteoarthritis initiative releases first data. National Institutes of Health; 2006. Available at: http://www.nih.gov/news/pr/aug2006/niams-01.htm. Accessed February 15, 2010.
51. Leonhardt D. America's sea of red ink was years in the making. New York Times 2009. Available at: http://www.nytimes.com/2009/06/10/business/economy/10leonhardt.html. Accessed February 15, 2010.
52. Brief analysis: President Obama's FY 2010 budget. Majority Staff, Senate Budget Committee; 2009. Available at: http://budget.senate.gov/democratic/statements/2009/Obama%20FY%202010%20Budget%20Brief%20Analysis_022709.pdf. Accessed February 15, 2010.
53. The budget and economic outlook: an update (August 2009). Congressional Budget Office; 2009. Available at: http://www.cbo.gov/ftpdocs/105xx/doc10521/08-25-BudgetUpdate.pdf. Accessed February 15, 2010.
54. Centers for Medicare and Medicaid Services. Updated and extended national health expenditure projections 2010–2019. Available at: http://www.cms.hhs.gov/NationalHealthExpendData/downloads/NHE_Extended_Projections.pdf. 2009. Accessed February 15, 2010.
55. Annual Report of the boards of trustees federal hospital insurance and federal supplementary medical insurance trust funds. Available at: http://www.cms.hhs.gov/ReportsTrustFunds/downloads/tr2009.pdf. 2009. Accessed February 15, 2010.
56. Health care reform: alternative perspectives. Harvard Medical School Symposium 2010; Harvard Joseph B. Martin Amphitheater. Attended by William H. Gruber.
57. Lee T, Mongan J. Chaos and organization in health care. Cambridge (MA): The MIT Press; 2009.
58. Kenney C. The best practice: how the new quality movement is transforming medicine. (F.W. Cleve Killingsworth). New York: Public Affairs; 2008.
59. Berwick DM, Nolan TW, Whittington J. The triple aim: care, health, and cost. Health Aff 2008;27(3):759–69.
60. Starr P. Fighting the wrong health care battle. New York Times 2009. Available at: http://www.nytimes.com/2009/11/29/opinion/29starr.html. Accessed February 15, 2010.
61. Swensen SJ, Meyer GS, Nelson EC, et al. Cottage industry to postindustrial care — the revolution in health care delivery. N Engl J Med 2010. Available at: http://healthcarereform.nejm.org/?p=2836&query=home. Accessed February 15, 2010.
62. Porter M. Competitive advantage. New York: The Free Press; 1985. p. 33–4.
63. Scholle SH. Developing and testing measures of patient-centered care. New York: Commonwealth Fund; 2006. Available at: http://www.commonwealthfund.org/Content/Spotlights/2006/Developing-and-Testing-Measures-of-Patient-Centered-Care.aspx. Accessed February 15, 2010.
64. Arnst C. The family doctor: a remedy for health-care costs. Bus Week 2009:34–7.
65. Fisher ES. Building a medical neighborhood for the medical home. N Engl J Med 2008;359(12):1202–12.
66. Smith MD. Disruptive innovation: can health care learn from other industries? A conversation with Clayton M. Christensen. Health Affairs-web exclusive. Available at: http://content.healthaffairs.org/cgi/content/abstract/hlthaff.26.3.w288. Accessed February 15, 2010
67. The patient centered medical home: history, seven core features, evidence and transformational change. Robert Graham Center; 2007. Available at: http://www.adfammed.org/documents/grahamcentermedicalhome.pdf. Accessed February 15, 2010.

68. Hackbarth G, Reischauer R, Mutti A. Collective accountability for medical care — toward bundled Medicare payments. N Engl J Med 2008;359:3–5.

69. Iglehart JK. No place like home – testing a new model of care delivery. N Engl J Med 2008;359(12):1200–2.

70. Browser BA. Pa. Hospitals Test 'Warranty' on Patient Care Transcript. Newshour with Jim Lehrer. PBS 2009.

71. Oldest baby boomers turn 60. US Census Bureau; 2006. Available at: http://www.census.gov/Press-Release/www/releases/archives/facts_for_features_special_editions/006105.html. Accessed February 15, 2010.

72. Agency for Health Care Policy and Research. Managing osteoarthritis: helping the elderly maintain function and mobility. Research in action. Rockville (MD): AHRQ Publication; 2002. Available at: http://www.ahrq.gov/research/osteoria/osteoria.htm. Accessed February 15, 2010.

73. Mango P, Riefberg V. Health savings accounts: making patients better consumers. McKinsey on health care. The McKinsey Quarterly 2005. Available at: http://www.mckinseyquarterly.com/Health_savings_accounts_Making_patients_better_consumers_1567. Accessed February 15, 2010.

74. Grunwald M. How to cut health-care costs: less care, more data. Time Magazine 2009. Available at: http://www.time.com/time/politics/article/0,8599,1905340,00.html. Accessed Feburary 15, 2010.

75. Arnst C. 10 ways to cut health-care costs right now: employers and hospitals don't have to wait for Congress to address inefficiences and waste. Bus Week 2009. Available at: http://www.businessweek.com/magazine/content/09_47/b4156034717852.htm. Accessed Feburary 15, 2010.

Strength Training in Older Adults: The Benefits for Osteoarthritis

Nancy Latham, PhD, PT[a],*, Chiung-ju Liu, PhD, OTR[b]

KEYWORDS

- Strength training • Older adults • Osteoarthritis
- Exercise training

Muscle weakness is a common impairment in older adults,[1,2] and osteoarthritis (OA) is one of the most frequently occurring chronic conditions in older people.[3] It therefore is not surprising that these conditions frequently coexist in the elderly. Skeletal muscles produce all voluntary human movement. Changes in properties and performance of muscles can profoundly affect an older person's ability to walk and function independently.[4–6] Loss of muscle strength might be particularly problematic for older persons with OA who have pain, stiffness, and mechanical changes to a joint that complicate their ability to mobilize and make them particularly vulnerable to small changes in their physical status.

Strength training has been the focus of a great deal of recent clinical research in many populations, including older adults and people with OA.[7–13] Although the benefits of strength training have been well explored in reviews focused on both populations, there has been little attention paid to the benefits and risks of strength training when undertaken by older people who have OA. In addition to being weaker, older people are more likely to have more advanced OA, including more severe pain and biomechanical changes to the joint, which might change their response to exercise training.

MUSCLE WEAKNESS IN OLDER ADULTS

Most adults attain their peak muscle strength in their mid-20s and maintain this level of strength relatively well until the sixth decade.[14] By age 80, strength declines on

[a] Health and Disability Research Institute, Boston University School of Public Health, 5TW, 715 Albany Street, Boston, MA, USA
[b] Department of Occupational Therapy, School of Health and Rehabilitation Sciences, Indiana University, 1140 West Michigan Street, CF 303, Indianapolis, IN 46202, USA
* Corresponding author.
E-mail address: nlatham@bu.edu

Clin Geriatr Med 26 (2010) 445–459
doi:10.1016/j.cger.2010.03.006
0749-0690/10/$ – see front matter © 2010 Elsevier Inc. All rights reserved.

geriatric.theclinics.com

average to almost half that of a young adult.[15] This decline in strength is consistent across muscle groups and all types of measurements—isometric strength (the limb does not move), concentric strength (the muscle shortens), eccentric strength (a lengthening contraction occurs), and strength measured isokinetically (at a fixed speed).[1,16]

In addition to a reduction in muscle strength, studies have shown enormous declines in muscle mass with age. One study found that the muscle mass of 80 year olds was 40% less than that of people in their 20s.[17] The loss of muscle strength and mass that occurs with age was given the name, *sarcopenia*, by Rosenberg[18] in 1989, from the Greek, *poverty of flesh*.

The New Mexico Elder Health Survey, involving 883 people, is the most comprehensive study to date of the prevalence of sarcopenia in older people.[19] This study defined sarcopenia as a loss of muscle mass of greater than 2 SDs below the mean appendicular muscle mass for healthy young adults. Among those aged 60 to 70 years, the prevalence of sarcopenia was approximately 17% for men and approximately 24% for women. Above age 80, the figure rose to 53% to 58% for men and 43% to 60% for women. Although these findings need to be confirmed in other populations, the high prevalence of sarcopenia in this study suggests that sarcopenia is a common disorder among older people.

MUSCLE WEAKNESS IN OA

Muscle weakness, particularly of the knee extensors, is common in people with OA[7,20] and has been consistently shown associated with an increased risk of functional limitations and disability.[20,21] One cohort study found lower-limb strength a stronger predictor of functional limitations than radiographic severity or knee pain.[21]

The nature of the cause-effect relationship between muscle weakness and OA is complex and has been widely debated. Although strength probably declines in people with OA as a secondary result of reduced activity, there is also evidence that muscle weakness directly contributes to the development and progression of OA.[20] Muscle strength seems to have a protective effect against the disability associated with progressing OA. In a longitudinal study that monitored a cohort of women for 6 years who had no functional limitations at baseline, knee extensor strength was protective against the development of functional limitations associated with OA.[22]

BENEFITS OF STRENGTH TRAINING

In older adults, there is now strong evidence from randomized controlled trials (RCTs) that even in the oldest old, muscle strength can be increased with a strength training program that uses a progressive overload.[12,13] There is also evidence that strength training improves mobility (ie, increased gait speed), simple functional tasks (ie, standing up from a chair), and self-rated daily function in older adults.[13] Although the effects of strength training are large, the impact on function and disability is more modest.

There are also many RCTs that support the benefits of exercise in general and strength training in particular in people with OA. Recent systematic reviews and guidelines have summarized the evidence for the effectiveness of strength training in people with OA and have found that strength training has a significant benefit in improving strength and function and in reducing pain.[9–11] These reviews have also found, however, that the reductions in pain and improvements in function are modest.

STRENGTH TRAINING BY OLDER ADULTS WITH OA

Although the positive benefits of strength training in the general population of older adults suggest that it would be beneficial for older people with OA, there are reasons to think that this might not be the case. Because OA is a painful musculoskeletal condition, it is possible that strength training might cause stress on the joints, which could exacerbate pain and result in decreased function and mobility. The biomechanical changes to the joint that occur with OA also have the potential to contribute to different responses to and risk factors from strength training.

No systematic review has focused specifically on strength training in older adults with OA. This review explores the evidence from all identified RCTs of people with OA undertaking strength training to determine the strength of the evidence to answer several questions. These questions are

- Does strength training improve strength and function and reduce pain in older people with OA?
- Are there differences in the effect of strength training in older adults with OA compared with the general population of older people?

There are other important questions about the benefits of strength training for older people with OA. Although there are inadequate data to allow a meta-analysis, the current evidence from RCTs is explored to determine whether or not the design of the strength training program influences their response to strength training.

SYSTEMATIC REVIEW METHODS
Criteria for Including Studies

This review includes only RCTs that provide the highest level of evidence of treatment efficacy. Because the focus of this review is on older adults, only studies where the participants had a mean age of 65 or above in the overall group or in the progressive resistance training (PRT) group were included. This review did not include exercise programs in which there was not a treatment arm where the subjects received only PRT. Because of these criteria, all studies where the intervention group received exercise programs that combined different types of exercise training (eg, aerobic and strength training) were excluded. This review also only included strength training programs that used PRT, because strength training programs that do not use this approach might be less effective. For this review, PRT was defined as strength training in which the overload increases during the training program to maintain or increase the intensity of the program.

Identifying Studies

To identify studies, the authors searched the Cochrane Bone, Joint and Muscle Trauma Group Specialized Register; the Cochrane Central Register of Controlled Trials; MEDLINE; Embase; CINAHL; SPORTDiscus; PEDro, the Physiotherapy Evidence Database; and Digital Dissertations (now ProQuest Dissertations and Theses) for all RCTs of strength training in older adults. Specific searches for OA exercise trials were conducted. Reference lists from other reviews and guidelines that summarized the evidence for strength training by people with OA were also reviewed. No language restrictions were applied.

The authors reviewed the titles, descriptors, or abstracts identified from all literature searches to identify potentially relevant trials for full review. A copy of the full text of all trials that seemed potentially suitable for the review was obtained. The authors used previously defined inclusion criteria to select the trials. Data were extracted for lower-extremity leg strength, pain, and self-rated function outcomes. Information about the study methods, subject characteristics, exercise program, adverse events, and exercise adherence was also recorded.

Data Synthesis

When adequate data were provided for the outcomes of lower-limb extensor strength, pain, or function, the results from each study were entered into the database and combined. Data synthesis was performed using MetaView in Review Manager, version 5.0. Standardized units (ie, standardized mean differences [SMDs]) were created to allow the pooling of outcomes using different units and 95% CIs were calculated. Random effects models were used for all analyses.

META-ANALYSIS RESULTS
Summary of Included Studies

A total of 8 studies were included in this review (**Table 1**).[23–30] Most studies that were not included in this review were excluded because the mean age was below 65 or the study included participants younger than 50; the exercise program included more types of exercises than PRT alone (eg, PRT and aerobic training).

All of the studies focused on people with knee OA, with one study including people with hip and knee OA.[25] The size of the studies ranged from 20 to 295 people.

The number of exercises included in the program varied from 1 exercise to 9. Most of the exercise programs were conducted at a moderate to high intensity. All of the programs had participants exercise 3 times per week, except in the study by Lim and colleagues,[26] where people exercised 5 times per week. The duration of the programs ranged from 6 to 72 weeks. In 3 studies, participants exercised only in a gym setting, 1 study used only home-based training, and 4 studies used a combination of home-based and gym-based training. A wide variety of equipment was used, including Thera-Bands, cuff weights, and isokinetic dynamometers.

In the study by Lim and colleagues,[26] the subjects were divided into 2 groups before randomization, people with neutral knee alignment and people with more varus malalignment. Because these groups were separately randomized, they were treated as 2 different studies for the purpose of the meta-analysis.

Effect of Strength Training on Strength and Function in Older People with OA

PRT improves strength in older adults with OA. The effect size for the impact that strength training has on leg extensor muscle strength of older adults with OA was moderate and the effect was statistically significant (**Fig. 1**), with an SMD of 0.33 (95% CI, 0.12, 0.54).

This review also found that strength training significantly improves function in older people with OA (**Figs. 2** and **3**). The effect of strength training on function was almost identical to the effect size found for strength, with an SMD of 0.33 (95% CI, 0.18, 0.49), which is statistically significant.

Pain decreased in people who participated in PRT. This effect was negative, indicating a reduction in pain, with an SMD of −0.35 (95% CI, −0.52, −0.18).

Comparison of Outcomes between Older People with and without OA

To compare the effects of strength training in older people with and without OA, newly identified trials were added to a database that included all previously identified trials of PRT in older people. As described elsewhere, this database includes trials of healthy older adults as well as older people with a variety of medical conditions.[13]

These analyses found that the studies of older adults that were not specifically focused on older people with OA had a much larger effect on strength than the

OA-specific studies (**Table 2**). When the OA-specific studies were excluded, the effect size for strength was 0.88 (95% CI, 0.7, 1.05), which is significantly lower than the strength estimate for older people with OA.

In contrast, the studies of strength training in the general population of older people had only a small effect on function (see **Table 2**). When the OA-specific studies were removed from the analysis, the effect of strength training on function was no longer statistically significant, with an effect size of 0.07 (95% CI, −0.02, 0.17). In contrast, the OA-specific studies had a moderate effect on function, which was significantly different from the small functional effect in the non–OA-specific studies.

DESIGN OF TRAINING PROGRAMS

From a clinical perspective, questions about the optimal design of a strength training program are important. There are fewer studies that have randomized comparisons of different strength training approaches in older adults with OA, so meta-analytic comparisons are not possible. Two studies with randomized comparisons of different strength training approaches are summarized later. Because so few studies exist in this area, the search was broadened to include studies where the mean age of participants was 60 or above.

High- Versus Low-Moderate–Intensity Strength Training

There has been debate about the most appropriate exercise intensity for strength training programs for people with OA. Larger training effects are usually seen when people participate in high-intensity strength training, but there is concern that a large overload might increase pain and joint stress in people with OA. Jan and colleagues[31] conducted an RCT that compared high-intensity and low-intensity training in people with knee OA. The investigators stated that their original intent had been to have people exercising at an intensity of 80% of 1 repetition maximum (1RM), but they found in pilot testing that 7 of 10 subjects were unable to complete the exercises at this intensity because of pain. Therefore, high-intensity training was conducted at 60% of 1RM with 3 sets of 8 repetitions and low-intensity training was set at 10% 1RM with 10 sets of 15 repetitions. After 8 weeks of training, both exercise groups had significantly reduced pain and improved function compared with the control group, but there were no significant differences in these outcomes between the high- and low-intensity training groups. No adverse events were reported.

Dynamic Versus Isometric Resistance Training

Topp and colleagues[30] compared a dynamic resistance training program where the exercises were performed through the range of motion using Thera-Band to an isometric training program where the joint did not move as the subjects generated muscle tension against the maximum-resistance Thera-Band while the joint angle did not change. After 16 weeks of training, both groups had improvements in function and pain compared with the control group, but the improvements were not significantly different between the 2 treatment groups.

DISCUSSION

This review found that strength training is beneficial to older people with OA. Older adults in the strength training group had significant improvements in strength and function and reductions in pains. All of these outcomes had a moderate effect size.

These findings are consistent with what is known about the effect of strength training in the general older adult population and in the general population of people

Table 1
Characteristics of included studies

Study ID	Sample Size	Mean Age	Intervention	Control	Exercise Adherence	OA Group
Schilke et al, 1996[29]	20	65	Type of ex: 1 LL Equipment: isokinetic dynamometer Intensity: high Frequency: 3× pw Reps/sets: 5/6 Duration: 8 weeks Setting: gym	Usual activities	NR	Knee OA
Ettinger et al, 1997[24]	295 (in PRT vs control)	68	Type of ex: 4 UL, 4 LL, 1 Tr Equipment: cuff weights, dumbbells Intensity: moderate to high Frequency: 3× pw Reps/sets: 12/2 Duration: 78 weeks Setting: facility-based group for 3 months, then home-based for 15 months	Health education program	70% at 18 Months	Knee OA
Maurer et al, 1999[27]	113	66.3	Type of ex: 1 LL Equipment: isokinetic dynamometer Intensity: high Frequency: 3× pw Reps/sets: 3 reps at 3 speeds (total 9 reps) in 3 sets Duration: 8 weeks Setting: gym	4 classes on OA education and self-management	NR	Knee OA

Study	N	Age	Intervention	Control	Adherence	Condition
Baker et al, 2001[23]	46	68	Type of ex: 2 functional exercises (squats and step-ups), 5 LL isotonic exercises Equipment: Velcro ankle weights Intensity: initially low, progressed to hard Frequency: 3× pw Reps/sets: 12/2 Duration: 16 weeks Setting: home based	Given nutrition info, 7 home visits over 16 weeks, kept food logs 3/14 days	84%	Knee OA
Topp et al, 2002[30]	35	65.6	Type of Ex: 6 LL for 30 minutes Equipment: Thera-Band Intensity: mild fatigue after 8RM Frequency: 3× pw (2 at home 1 at gym) Reps/sets: increasing reps and sets every week and then reached 12 reps/3 sets at week 9 Duration: 16 weeks Setting: home and gym	No intervention	NR	Knee OA
Foley et al, 2003[25]	70	69.8	Type of ex: 1 UE/4 LL Equipment: weighted gaiters Intensity: 10RM Frequency: 3× pw Reps/sets: not reported Duration: 6 weeks Setting: gym	Telephone calls to record any changes in their condition	75%	Hip or knee OA

(continued on next page)

Table 1
(continued)

Study ID	Sample Size	Mean Age	Intervention	Control	Exercise Adherence	OA Group
Mikesky et al, 2006[28]	221	69.4	Type of ex: 2 UL/2 LL Equipment: CYBEX machines at gym; elastic bands at home Intensity: 8–10RM Frequency: 3× pw Duration: 1 year Setting: gym and home	Flexibility exercise group: flexibility ex, 3× pw	59% Gym 56% Home	Knee OA
Lim et al, 2008[26] malaligned	52	67.2	Type of ex: 5 LL Equipment: Thera-Band and cuff weights Intensity: 10RM Frequency: 5× pw Reps/sets: initially 2 sets of 10 reps, progressed to 3 sets of 10 reps Duration: 12 weeks Setting: gym and home	No intervention	89%	Medial knee OA
Lim et al, 2008[26] neutral	55	64.1	Same program as Lim et al, 2008 malaligned	No intervention	86%	Medial knee OA

Abbreviations: ex, exercise; LL, lower limb; NR, not reported; reps, repetitions; Tr, trunk; UL, upper limb; × pw, times per week.

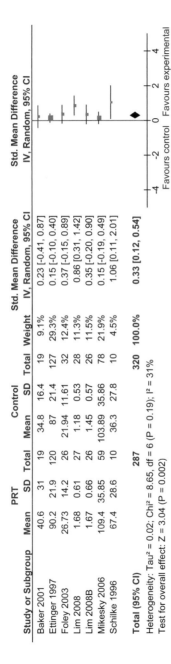

Study or Subgroup	PRT Mean	SD	Total	Control Mean	SD	Total	Weight	Std. Mean Difference IV, Random, 95% CI	Std. Mean Difference IV, Random, 95% CI
Baker 2001	40.6	31	19	34.8	16.4	19	9.1%	0.23 [-0.41, 0.87]	
Ettinger 1997	90.2	21.9	120	87	21.4	127	29.3%	0.15 [-0.10, 0.40]	
Foley 2003	26.73	14.2	26	21.94	11.61	32	12.4%	0.37 [-0.15, 0.89]	
Lim 2008	1.68	0.61	27	1.18	0.53	28	11.3%	0.86 [0.31, 1.42]	
Lim 2008B	1.67	0.66	26	1.45	0.57	26	11.5%	0.35 [-0.20, 0.90]	
Mikesky 2006	109.4	35.85	59	103.89	35.86	78	21.9%	0.15 [-0.19, 0.49]	
Schilke 1996	67.4	28.6	10	36.3	27.8	10	4.5%	1.06 [0.11, 2.01]	
Total (95% CI)			287			320	100.0%	0.33 [0.12, 0.54]	

Heterogeneity: Tau^2 = 0.02; Chi^2 = 8.65, df = 6 (P = 0.19); I^2 = 31%
Test for overall effect: Z = 3.04 (P = 0.002)

Favours control   Favours experimental

Fig. 1. Forest plot of leg extensor strength in trials of strength training by older adults with OA. Mean and SD are based on the final scores for each outcome measure in the PRT and control groups. Total refers to the sample size in each group for each outcome. The sample size is used to weight the contribution of each study to the overall estimate of treatment effect. The total SMD indicates what the overall effect size and the associated CI are for this estimate. The test of statistical significance is provided by the test for overall effect and the associated P value, which is shown to the far left of the figure.

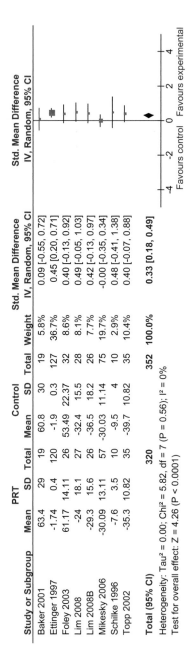

Study or Subgroup	PRT			Control			Weight	Std. Mean Difference IV, Random, 95% CI
	Mean	SD	Total	Mean	SD	Total		
Baker 2001	63.4	29	19	60.8	30	19	5.8%	0.09 [-0.55, 0.72]
Ettinger 1997	-1.74	0.4	120	-1.9	0.3	127	36.7%	0.45 [0.20, 0.71]
Foley 2003	61.17	14.11	26	53.49	22.37	32	8.6%	0.40 [-0.13, 0.92]
Lim 2008	-24	18.1	27	-32.4	15.5	28	8.1%	0.49 [-0.05, 1.03]
Lim 2008B	-29.3	15.6	26	-36.5	18.2	26	7.7%	0.42 [-0.13, 0.97]
Mikesky 2006	-30.09	13.11	57	-30.03	11.14	75	19.7%	-0.00 [-0.35, 0.34]
Schilke 1996	-7.6	3.5	10	-9.5	4	10	2.9%	0.48 [-0.41, 1.38]
Topp 2002	-35.3	10.82	35	-39.7	10.82	35	10.4%	0.40 [-0.07, 0.88]
Total (95% CI)			320			352	100.0%	0.33 [0.18, 0.49]

Heterogeneity: Tau² = 0.00; Chi² = 5.82, df = 7 (P = 0.56); I² = 0%
Test for overall effect: Z = 4.26 (P < 0.0001)

Fig. 2. Forest plot of function in trials of strength training by older adults with OA.

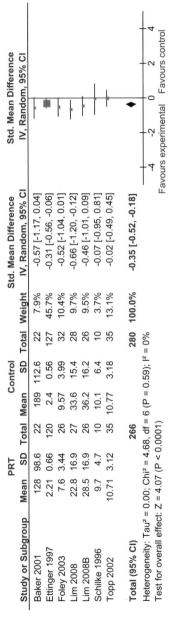

Study or Subgroup	PRT Mean	SD	Total	Control Mean	SD	Total	Weight	Std. Mean Difference IV, Random, 95% CI
Baker 2001	128	98.6	22	189	112.6	22	7.9%	-0.57 [-1.17, 0.04]
Ettinger 1997	2.21	0.66	120	2.4	0.56	127	45.7%	-0.31 [-0.56, -0.06]
Foley 2003	7.6	3.44	26	9.57	3.99	32	10.4%	-0.52 [-1.04, 0.01]
Lim 2008	22.8	16.9	27	33.6	15.4	28	9.7%	-0.66 [-1.20, -0.12]
Lim 2008B	28.5	16.9	26	36.2	16.2	26	9.5%	-0.46 [-1.01, 0.09]
Schilke 1996	9.7	4.7	10	10.1	6.4	10	3.7%	-0.07 [-0.95, 0.81]
Topp 2002	10.71	3.12	35	10.77	3.18	35	13.1%	-0.02 [-0.49, 0.45]
Total (95% CI)			266			280	100.0%	-0.35 [-0.52, -0.18]

Heterogeneity: Tau² = 0.00; Chi² = 4.68, df = 6 (P = 0.59); I² = 0%
Test for overall effect: Z = 4.07 (P < 0.0001)

Favours experimental   Favours control

Std. Mean Difference IV, Random, 95% CI

Fig. 3. Forest plot of pain in trials of strength training by older adults with OA.

Table 2
Comparison of strength and functional outcomes between older adults with and without OA

Outcome	Comparison	N	Effect Size (95% CI)
Strength	All older adults	3166	0.83 (0.67, 0.98)
	Excluding OA-specific studies	2559	0.88 (0.7, 1.05)
	Including only OA-specific studies	607	0.33 (0.12, 0.54)
Function	All older adults	2279	0.15 (0.07, 0.23)
	Excluding OA-specific studies	1607	0.07 (−0.02, 0.17)
	Including only OA-specific studies	672	0.33 (0.18, 0.49)

with OA, where strength training has been found to improve muscle strength and function.[11,13,23] The effect on strength was smaller than that found by Fransen and McConnell[9] in a Cochrane review of knee OA, which found an effect size of 0.53 (95% CI, 0.79, 0.27), although the CIs overlap. It is not clear why the results were different in this review. It is possible that the studies that included younger people with OA were more likely to use the highest intensity of training or had other differences in the program, but such differences in the training programs are not apparent in the study descriptions. It is also possible that the older people's muscles were slightly less responsive overall or slower to respond to the training stimulus. Finally, it is possible that adherence to the exercise program was lower in older people with OA, but this cannot be confirmed because adherence was poorly recorded or not recorded at all in many of these trials.

This review found a difference in the magnitude of the effect on strength and function between studies with a general older adult population and OA-specific studies of older people. In the general older adult population, strength training has a large effect on strength and a much smaller, barely significant, effect on function. This is perhaps not surprising, because the intervention is targeting muscle, so the direct impact is on strength, whereas many factors can contribute to late-life functional problems. In OA, the effect on strength, function, and pain was a moderate size, and almost an identical effect size across the 3 outcomes. These findings suggest that although strength training is beneficial for all older adults, it has a much larger functional impact on people with OA, and all of the improvements in muscle strength are directly translated into improvements in function. One reason for this could be that the impairments that limit function in older people with OA are more narrowly focused, and muscle weakness is a primary contributor to pain and functional problems in OA. When older people with OA participate in strength training, the training directly targets one of the main barriers to their functional performance.

It is not clear why the strength gains in people with OA were smaller than those in the general older adult population. Given the larger strength gains observed in the general older adults studies, it would seem that larger strength gains are possible to achieve in older adults exercisers. It is possible that if strength gains could be increased in older people with OA, perhaps by changes to the type, intensity, or duration of training or by ensuring maximal adherence to the training, there might also be additional improvements in function and reductions in pain beyond the moderate effects currently seen.

A major limitation of this review is that no appropriate RCTs were identified that explored the effects of strength training on older adults with hip or upper-limb OA. Any studies that were identified could not be included because they focused on a younger population, did not use an RCT design, or used combined exercise training or a non-PRT approach. Studies in these groups of OA patients are needed.

There are also limited randomized data available about the comparative effectiveness of different strength programs or even the relative effectiveness of different training approaches. The existing evidence suggests that there are few differences in outcomes when different training approaches are used. In particular, Jan and colleagues found no significant differences in strength and functional outcomes between high- and low-intensity training groups. Caution is needed, however, in interpreting these findings because the studies comparing training intensity or approaches have all had a short duration of follow-up so true training effects might not have occurred. They also have small sample sizes and, therefore, might have failed to detect real differences that exist between the treatment groups because of a lack of statistical power.

The positive message from this review that should be communicated to older people with OA is that no matter how old they are, they will probably benefit in clinically important ways from participating in a strength training program, as long as it provides some consistent overload to their muscles as they exercise. The biggest challenge with any exercise program is maintaining long-term adherence, because the benefits of exercise diminish if people stop exercising. There is currently no evidence that one type of strength training program is superior to another as long as a program provides progressive overload, so older people should exercise at the intensity and location and using the equipment that they most prefer. Although not the focus of this review, aerobic training programs have been found to have a similar benefit to strength training in an RCT that had one of the largest sample sizes and longest follow-up of any trials in this area.[24] If people prefer aerobic exercise, this mode of exercise should also be used by older people with OA.

SUMMARY

Older adults with OA benefit from a strength training program that provides progressive overload to maintain intensity throughout the exercise program. Significant improvements in strength and function and pain reduction were seen when the data from 8 RCTs were synthesized, and there was a moderate effect size for all 3 outcomes.

Clinicians should encourage participation in exercise training programs, even in the oldest old with OA. There is no evidence that there is significantly decreased efficacy or increased risk of adverse events when older adults with OA participate in exercise programs compared with younger adults. People with OA should be reassured that it is unlikely to exacerbate their pain if performed using the appropriate methods and at the appropriate dose. The evidence suggests that it decreases pain in most older people.

More information is needed about the comparative effectiveness of different training approaches. Specifically, trials with adequate sample size and duration of follow-up are needed to comparing the effectiveness of different training intensities and types of strength training approaches. Current evidence suggests, however, that people can benefit from a wide variety of exercise programs, as long as the strength training program provides a progressive overload. Older people with OA should, therefore, select the type and style of strength training that best fits their lifestyle. Long-term adherence is required to maintain the benefits of strength training, and studies to increase understanding of the best way to achieve long-term compliance with exercise programs in this population would be useful.

Finally, more evidence is needed about the benefits of strength training for older people with OA of the hip and upper limb. Current findings are almost completely based on studies of people with knee OA.

ACKNOWLEDGMENTS

The authors wish to acknowledge the contributions of Craig Anderson, Derrick Bennett, and Caroline Stretton who were involved in the first Cochrane systematic review of strength training in older adults. They also wish to thank Kira Wilke and Amy Vertal for their assistance in the preparation of this manuscript. Dr Latham was supported by the Boston Pepper Center Research Career and Development Core, which is funded through the National Institute of Health.

REFERENCES

1. Vandervoort A. Effects of ageing on human neuromuscular function: implications for exercise. Can J Sport Sci 1992;17(3):178–84.
2. Brooks SV, Faulkner JA. Skeletal muscle weakness in old age: underlying mechanisms. Med Sci Sports Exerc 1994;26(4):432–9.
3. Seeman TE, Merkin SS, Crimmins EM, et al. Disability trends among older Americans: National Health and Nutrition Examination surveys, 1988–1994 and 1999–2004. Am J Public Health 2010;100:100–7.
4. Buchner DM, de Lateur BJ. The importance of skeletal muscle strength to physical function in older adults. Ann Behav Med. 1991;13:91–8.
5. Buchner DM, Larson EB, Wagner EH, et al. Evidence for a non-linear relationship between leg strength and gait speed. Age Ageing 1996;25:386–91.
6. Jette A, Assmann S, Rooks D, et al. Interrelationships among disablement concepts. J Gerontol A Biol Sci Med Sci 1998;53(5):M395–404.
7. Baker K, McAlindon T. Exercise for knee osteoarthritis. Curr Opin Rheumatol 2000;12:456–63.
8. Singh MA. Exercise comes of age: rationale and recommendations for a geriatric exercise prescription. J Gerontol A Biol Sci Med Sci 2002;57(5):M262–82.
9. Fransen M, McConnell S. Exercise for osteoarthritis of the knee. Cochrane Database Syst Rev 2008;4:CD004376.
10. Fransen M, McConnell S, Bell M. Exercise for osteoarthritis of the hip or knee. Cochrane Database Syst Rev 2003;3:CD004286.
11. Lange AK, Vanwanseele B, Fiatarone Singh MA. Strength training for treatment of osteoarthritis of the knee: a systematic review. Arthritis Rheum 2008;59(10):1488–94.
12. Latham N, Bennet DA, Stretton CM, et al. A systematic review of progressive resistance strength training in older adults. J Gerontol A Biol Sci Med Sci 2004;59(1):48–61.
13. Liu CJ, Latham NK. Progressive resistance strength training for improving physical function in older adults. Cochrane Database Syst Rev 2009;3:CD002759.
14. Lindle RS, Metter EJ, Lynch NA, et al. Age and gender comparisons of muscle strength in 654 women and men aged 20–93 yr. J Appl Phys 1997;83(5):1581–7.
15. Doherty T, Vandervoort A, Brown W. Effects of ageing on the motor unit: a brief review. Can J Appl Physiol 1993;18(4):331–58.
16. Hughes VA, Frontera WR, Wood M, et al. Longitudinal muscle strength changes in older adults: influence of muscle mass, physical activity and health. J Gerontol A Biol Sci Med Sci 2001;56(5):B209–17.
17. Lexell J, Taylor CC, Sjostrom M. What is the cause of the ageing atrophy? Total number, size and proportion of different fiber types studied in whole vastus lateralis muscle from 15- to 83-year-old men. J Neurol Sci 1988;84(2–3):275–94.
18. Rosenberg IH. Summary comments. Am J Clin Nutr 1989;50:1231–3.

19. Baumgartner RN, Koehler KM, Gallagher D, et al. Epidemiology of sarcopenia among the elderly in New Mexico. Am J Epidemiol 1998;147(8):755–63.
20. Slemenda C, Brandt KD, Heilman DK, et al. Quadriceps weakness and osteoarthritis of the knee. Ann Intern Med 1997;127:97–104.
21. McAlindon TE, Cooper AC, Kirwan JR, et al. Determinants of disability in osteoarthritis of the knee. Ann Rheum Dis 1993;52:258–62.
22. Ling SM, Xue QL, Simonsick EM, et al. Transitions to mobility difficulty associated with lower extremity osteoarthritis in high functioning older women: longitudinal data from the Women's Health and Aging Study II. Arthritis Rheum. 2006;55: 256–63.
23. Baker KR, Nelson ME, Felson DT, et al. The efficacy of home based progressive strength training in older adults with knee osteoarthritis: a randomized controlled trial. J Rheumatol 2001;28(7):1655–65.
24. Ettinger WH Jr, Burns R, Messier SP, et al. A randomized trial comparing aerobic exercise and resistance exercise with a health education program in older adults with knee osteoarthritis. The Fitness Arthritis and Seniors Trial (FAST). JAMA 1997;277:25–31.
25. Foley A, Halbert J, Hewitt T, et al. Does hydrotherapy improve strength and physical function in patients with osteoarthritis—a randomised controlled trial comparing a gym based and a hydrotherapy based strengthening programme. Ann Rheum Dis 2003;62(12):1162–7.
26. Lim BW, Hinman RS, Wrigley TV, et al. Does knee malalignment mediate the effects of quadriceps strengthening on knee adduction moment, pain and function in medial knee osteoarthritis? A randomized controlled trial. Arthritis Rheum 2008;59:943–51.
27. Maurer BT, Stern AG, Kinossian B, et al. Osteoarthritis of the knee: isokinetic quadriceps exercise versus an educational intervention. Arch Phys Med Rehabil 1999;80(10):1293–9.
28. Mikesky A, Mazzuca S, Brandt K, et al. Effects of strength training on the incidence and progression of knee osteoarthritis. Arthritis Care Res 2006;55(5): 690–9.
29. Schilke JM, Johnson GO, Housh TJ, et al. Effects of muscle-strength training on the functional status of patients with osteoarthritis of the knee joint. Nurse Res 1996;45(2):68–72.
30. Topp R, Woolley S, Hornyak J, et al. The effect of dynamic versus isometric resistance training on pain and functioning among adults with osteoarthritis of the knee. Arch Phys Med Rehabil 2002;83(9):1187–95.
31. Jan MH, Lin JJ, Liau JJ, et al. Investigation of the clinical effects of high- and low-resistance trainign for patients with knee osteoarthritis: a randomized controlled trial. Phys Ther 2008;88:427–36.

Diet and Exercise for Obese Adults with Knee Osteoarthritis

Stephen P. Messier, PhD

KEYWORDS

- Obesity • Knee osteoarthritis • Degenerative joint disease
- Exercise • Weight loss

First documented in 1945,[1] numerous studies have verified the strong association between obesity and knee osteoarthritis (OA). Leach and colleagues[2] found that 83% of their female subjects with knee OA were obese compared with 42% of the control group. Coggon and colleagues,[3] in a case-controlled study of 675 matched pairs, determined the risk of knee OA in people with a body mass index (BMI) of 30 kg/m^2 or higher was 6.8 times that of normal weight controls and increased exponentially as obesity increased (**Fig. 1**). Felson and colleagues[4] showed that a 5.1-kg loss in body mass over a 10-year period reduced the odds of developing OA by more than 50%. Ettinger and colleagues[5] examined the effects of comorbid diseases on disability and found that those with a BMI higher than 30 kg/m^2 were 4.2 times more likely to have knee OA than persons with a BMI lower than 30 kg/m^2. Knee OA and obesity were each significantly associated with poorer physical function, with odds ratios of 4.3 and 1.7, respectively; when obesity was combined with knee OA the odds ratio increased to 9.8. Taken together, these studies indicate that obesity is a major risk factor for knee OA.

The most common location of OA is in the small joints of the hand. Unlike knee OA, the association between obesity and hand OA is not strong. Doherty and colleagues[6] reviewed the literature on hand OA and concluded that BMI and waist circumference were not risk factors, especially in older adults. Similarly, Kalichman and Kobyliansky[7] used an observational cross-sectional design to study 745 women with hand OA and saw no relationship between BMI or waist circumference and hand OA. The investigators suggested that obesity may be a mechanical rather than a systemic risk factor for OA. This would explain obesity's strong association with OA of weight-bearing joints.

Supported by National Institutes of Health grants 1R01AR052528-01 and M01-RR-0021.
Department of Health and Exercise Science, Wake Forest University, Winston-Salem, PO Box 7868, NC 27109, USA
E-mail address: messier@wfu.edu

Clin Geriatr Med 26 (2010) 461–477
doi:10.1016/j.cger.2010.05.001
0749-0690/10/$ – see front matter © 2010 Elsevier Inc. All rights reserved.

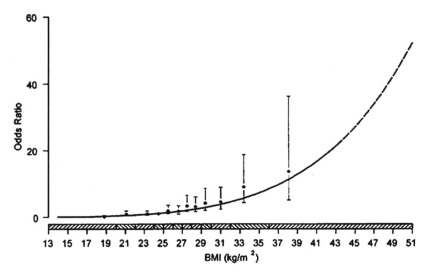

Fig. 1. Odds of knee OA (odds ratios and 95% confidence intervals) attributable to BMI (for 12 BMI categories of BMI). (*From* Coggon D, Reading I, Croft P, et al. Knee osteoarthritis and obesity. Int J Obes Relat Metab Disord 2001;25:622–7; with permission.)

IMPACT OF OBESITY ON FUNCTION AND GAIT

Increasing BMI has an adverse effect on balance, muscle strength, and gait, especially vertical ground reaction forces. The NHANES I and Epidemiologic Follow-up (NHEFS) studies revealed that obesity at baseline increased upper and lower body disability across 20 years of follow-up.[5,8] More recently, Jenkins[9] found that functional impairment in older adults increased as BMI increased. In the Cardiovascular Health Study, an adjusted odds ratio of 2.94 for self-reported mobility-related disability was found for those in the highest versus the lowest quintile of fat mass.[10]

As body weight increases there is an increase in both fat mass and fat-free mass.[11] The relationship between fat-free mass and BMI is stronger in males, suggesting that an increase in BMI in females is attributable predominately to an increase in fat mass. Although these data imply that obese people have greater strength than their nonobese counterparts, the opposite actually is true. Specifically, when strength is represented as a function of body weight, both obese males and females are weaker, irrespective of age.[12] In older adults aged 60 to 80 years, mean knee strength in obese males is 65% of body weight compared with 77% for controls, and 50% of body weight for obese females compared with 62% for nonobese females.

Muscle weakness in older adults is of great consequence. It is the second leading cause of falls in the elderly, accounting for 17% of all falls.[13] Falls are the leading cause of death by injury in older adults. Three-quarters of deaths attributable to falls occur in adults older than 65 years. Only one-half of those older adults hospitalized because of falls will be alive after 1 year. By 2030, deaths attributable to falls will reach 280,000 Americans annually.[14]

Falls occur because of a loss in balance; hence, it is common to use measures of balance to identify people who are more susceptible to falls. Kejonen and colleagues[15] found significant correlations between poor balance and high BMI in women, but not in men, once again suggesting that muscle weakness is a mediator of poor balance and falls. Within older adults with a BMI above 30 kg/m², Jadelis and colleagues[16] found that for a given amount of knee strength, the more severe the obesity, the worse the balance. This suggests that obesity, independent of strength, is a risk factor for poor balance and falls.

Plantar fasciitis and heel pain are commonly associated with obesity. In a case-controlled study, obese subjects were 5 times more likely to have heel pain than their nonobese counterparts with an odds ratio of 5.6.[17] Similarly, obese men and women exert greater plantar pressure during both standing and walking.[18–22] Hills and colleagues[19] found a significant correlation (r = 0.81) between midfoot peak pressure and BMI (**Fig. 2**). Gravante and colleagues[23] found greater midfoot weight-bearing area in obese men and women versus a control. The additional pressure on the medial longitudinal arch could have a detrimental effect on the plantar ligaments resulting in collapse. Considering that the medial longitudinal arch is critical in distributing loads to both the rearfoot and forefoot, it is not surprising that foot aliments are common among obese people.

Abnormal gait is also characteristic of obese people. Messier and colleagues[24] found that a severely overweight population walked with bilateral abducted forefeet or a more toed-out stance that was 276% greater than a normal weight group. Chodera and Levell[25] suggested that the feet have different functions, with the more abducted forefoot responsible for balance and the less abducted foot responsible for direction. In severely obese people, the amount of abduction is significantly greater in both feet relative to a normal weight control group, indicating a need for balance and suggesting that balance is more important than direction.[24]

In addition to the greater forefoot angles, severely obese people have more rearfoot motion.[24] More specifically, greater touchdown angle, more pronation range of motion, and a faster pronation velocity are typical of severely obese gait. This excessive rearfoot motion may cause injury and discomfort and has a negative effect on mobility.

Liu and Nigg[26] examined the effects of rigid and soft tissue mass on impact forces during running. They termed the soft tissue mass wobbling mass. Their spring-damper-mass model consisted of upper and lower body rigid and wobbling masses. A computer simulation found that upper body wobbling mass had no effect on impact forces, but had a strong influence on the propulsive peak. As upper body wobbling mass increased, vertical force propulsive peaks increased. In contrast, an increase in lower body wobbling mass showed a strong influence on impact peak forces. These

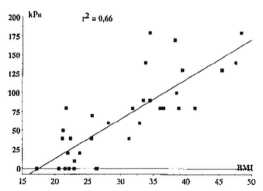

Fig. 2. Relationship between midfoot peak pressure and BMI. (*From* Hills AP, Hennig EM, McDonald M, et al. Plantar pressure differences between obese and non-obese adults: a biomechanical analysis. Int J Obes Relat Metab Disord 2001;25:1674–9; with permission.)

results suggest that obese individuals would exert greater forces during gait, because of their greater wobbling mass.

Empiric data support Liu and Nigg's model. Messier and colleagues[27] found a strong positive association between BMI and peak ground reaction forces ($r = 0.76$, $P = .0001$) in older adults with knee OA. This was also the case in a study by Browning and Kram,[28] who found that obese people exerted 60% greater vertical ground reaction forces compared with normal weight people (**Fig. 3**).

Obesity is also related to a fear of falling and injury risk.[29,30] Austin and colleagues[29] followed 1282 community-dwelling women aged 70 to 85 years for 3 years and found that fear of falling at baseline was independently associated with obesity, and obesity also was associated with the new-onset of fear of falling in women who were symptom free at baseline. In a sample of more than 42,000 adults, the odds of sustaining an injury were greater among those with excess weight. As BMI category increased from overweight ($25.0 \text{ kg/m}^2 \le \text{BMI} \le 29.9 \text{ kg/m}^2$) to class III obesity (BMI ≥ 40.0 kg/m^2), the odds of sustaining an injury, including those related to falls, rose from 15% to 48%.[30]

Obese adults make adjustments to help stabilize their larger mass and reduce fall risk. DeVita and Hortobagyi[31] compared obese and lean adults and noted that the obese group increased ankle torque during walking, but showed no difference in knee or hip torque. Specifically, the ankle plantar flexors act eccentrically to control the forward motion of the leg throughout stance, to stabilize body mass, and at toe-off, assist in propulsion. The greater mass in obese people requires more ankle plantar flexor torque to perform these tasks.

Obese people also try to reduce the load on the knee by shortening stride length and reducing the knee extensor torque. In an obese cohort, the greater the BMI, the shorter the stride length and the lower the knee joint extensor/flexor torque, with an actual shifting from an overall extensor torque to a dominant flexor torque at high BMIs. This switch results in knee stability being provided by the hamstrings rather than the quadriceps. In lean subjects, the relationships between BMI and stride length and knee torques do not exist, indicating that lower BMI values have little effect on gait.[31] In summary, during gait, obese adults exert greater forces than normal weight adults. As obesity worsens, this compensatory strategy increases, and minimizing

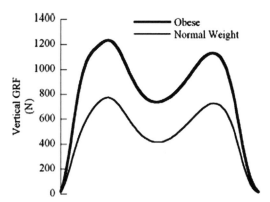

Fig. 3. Vertical ground reaction forces (GRF) during the stance phase of gait. Obese individuals exert 60% more vertical ground reaction force than normal-weight individuals. (*From* Browning RC, Kram R. Effects of obesity on the biomechanics of walking at different speeds. Med Sci Sports Exerc 2007;39:1632–41; with permission.)

these loads is attempted by shortening stride length. Taken together, these results suggest that adjusting gait mechanics without reducing body weight does not eliminate the detrimental effects obesity has on the lower extremity.

INFLAMMATION AND OA

Recent studies confirm that low-grade inflammation plays a pathophysiological role in OA. It may contribute to functional limitation, disease progression, and lower the pain threshold. One of our earlier studies showed that the inflammatory cytokine interleukin-1 beta (IL-1β) was present in the joint fluids of patients with OA.[32] IL-1β is believed to play a role in mediating joint inflammation and cartilage degradation in OA. Likewise, an inflammatory component associated with OA can be detected in the circulation, because serum concentrations of inflammatory markers such as cytokines (IL-6, tumor necrosis factor alpha [TNF-α]) and the acute-phase reactant C-reactive protein (CRP) are higher in persons with knee or hip OA compared with those without OA.[33–35] Longitudinal studies demonstrate that high serum levels of CRP and TNF-α predict increased radiographic progression of knee OA as much as 5 years later.[34,36,37] Moreover, a few studies, including one from our group,[38] associate OA severity and physical function with higher inflammatory markers in the blood.[39,40] Thus, severity, mobility, pain, stiffness, and radiographic progression are at least partly mediated by the level of chronic inflammation in patients with OA. Diffusion of cytokines from the synovial fluid into the cartilage could contribute to the cartilage matrix loss observed in OA by stimulating chondrocyte catabolic activity and inhibiting anabolic activity. The adipokine leptin increases synthesis of transforming growth factor beta (TGFβ) within the joint; TGFβ is a known stimulator of osteophyte formation.[41] Weight loss lowers serum leptin levels in subjects with OA and is related to improved function.[42]

EFFECTS OF WEIGHT LOSS

Weight loss reduces risk factors for symptomatic knee OA and lowers proinflammatory cytokines and adipokines thought to play a role in cartilage degradation. Our Arthritis, Diet, and Activity Promotion Trial (ADAPT)[43] diet groups achieved 5% weight loss over 18 months using a reduced-calorie diet with behavioral strategies, and the Physical Activity, Inflammation, and Body Composition Trial (PACT) pilot study achieved a 9% weight loss over 6 months in obese older adults with knee OA by combining a partial meal-replacement plan with accepted behavioral strategies.[44] Using a similar cohort and an intensive low-energy diet that achieved an 11% weight loss, Christensen and colleagues[45] found a threefold improvement in Western Ontario and McMaster Universities Arthritis Index function over an 8-week period compared with a control diet group who lost 4% of their body weight. Cognitive strategies were used to promote behavior change. A recent meta-analysis of 35 potential trials identified only 4 that met the investigators' inclusion criteria. From these 4 studies, they concluded that weight loss in patients with knee OA significantly reduces disability and that a weight loss of at least 10% would result in a moderate-to-large clinical effect.[46] Christensen and colleagues[45] concluded that weight loss should be the first-choice therapy for obese adults with knee OA.

Randomized clinical trials (RCTs) that examined weight loss in adults older than 65 reported no difference in mortality compared with groups that did not lose weight.[47,48] In contrast, randomization to weight reduction in the ADAPT trial decreased the risk of mortality by 50% (hazard rate ratio = 0.5, confidence interval [CI] = 0.3–1.0) over 8 years of follow-up (weight loss groups =15 deaths; non–weight loss groups = 30 deaths).[49] Diehr and colleagues[50] suggested that for the aged population, quality of life and years of healthy life may be more appropriate outcomes than mortality. However, the ADAPT follow-up mortality data provide new evidence for clinicians regarding the importance of intentional weight loss in older adults.

Loss of bone and muscle mass is a problem in weight-loss programs for older adults. Weight loss is associated with decreased bone-mineral density,[51,52] increased bone turnover,[52] and increased fracture rates.[53,54] Fiatarone Singh[55] noted that combining hypocaloric diets with aerobic exercise in older adults resulted in loss of lean mass that resistance training tended to offset. Janssen and colleagues[56] found no lean tissue loss when diet was combined with resistance or aerobic training in premenopausal women. In contrast, Wang and colleagues[57] found that a 6-month weight-loss intervention that incorporated partial meal replacements and aerobic and resistance exercises for older obese adults with knee OA resulted in an 8.1% weight loss of which 19.9% was lean mass. However, the exercise training improved knee-extensor strength by 37% compared with a 1% loss of strength in a weight-stable control group. These results show that intentional weight loss, when combined with aerobic and resistance exercise training, improves knee-extensor strength despite loss of lean body mass.

DIETARY WEIGHT LOSS INTERVENTIONS

Wadden and colleagues[58,59] note that achieving permanent weight loss in obese individuals is difficult. Successful weight loss and maintenance programs include behavioral change strategies, extended treatment, increased hours of intervention contact, adherence to a rigorous diet, participation in exercise, and inclusion of significant others.[60,61] Wing and colleagues[62] improved weight loss with increased treatment duration and intensity. Although maintaining weight loss is challenging, individual attention to coping strategies and increased intervention efforts during the maintenance phase have produced success. Approximately 80% of clients on moderate calorie restriction will remain in treatment for 20 weeks, and approximately 50% will lose 9.1 kg or more. An average weekly loss of 0.4 to 0.5 kg, with an average one-third regained 1 year after treatment is expected. Perri and colleagues[63] showed that a 13.2-kg weight loss was maintained by participants in a 20-week behavioral therapy program followed by an 18-week maintenance program with biweekly contact. Maintaining weight loss seems to require rigorous follow-up contacts. Esposito and colleagues[64] produced a 14.7% loss in body weight over a 2-year period in women following a moderate energy restricted diet of 1300 kcals per day for year 1 and 1500 kcals per day for year 2. This intervention used education, individualized goal setting, self-monitoring, and a structured exercise program.

The long-term effectiveness of low-fat and low-carbohydrate diets are currently under considerable debate. Meta-analyses have found them no more effective than a low-calorie diet in reducing weight and improving cardiovascular risk factors.[65,66] Increasingly popular meal-replacement diet drinks have been studied as a complement to reduced-calorie diets (termed partial meal-replacement diets). Heymsfield and colleagues[67] performed meta- and pooled analyses of 6 clinical trials that compared partial meal replacement to reduced calorie diet plans and found greater weight loss, reduced risk factors, and a lower drop-out rate with the partial meal-replacement plan, but the small number of trials limited conclusions.

In overweight and obese adults with knee OA, caloric restriction combined with an appropriate calorie distribution (15%–20% from protein; <30% from fat; 45%–60% from carbohydrate) should be the focus of any dietary intervention. Decreasing body weight will impact the osteoarthritis disease pathways by reducing the load on the knee and lowering proinflammatory cytokine activity.[68] An initial energy-intake deficit of 800 to 1000 kcals per day with a minimum intake of 1100 kcal for women and 1200 kcals for men would provide a safe and effective weight-loss plan.[68] A weight loss of 5% of body weight will reduce pain, improve function, and increase mobility.[43] Considering the potential effects of weight loss on the osteoarthritic process, a reduction in body weight of 2 to 3 times this magnitude (10%–15%) may slow disease progression.[68]

EFFECTS OF EXERCISE

The difficulty patients with knee OA have with activities of daily living often results in activity avoidance. Aerobic exercise is an effective nonpharmacologic treatment with medium effect sizes for improvements in pain and function (ES_{pooled} = 0.46–0.52).[69] Walking is the most common mode of aerobic exercise tested in the older, disabled population, although aquatic exercise has also proven effective in improving clinical symptoms.[70–74]

Several studies have shown that pain, physical function, and walking distance improve an average of 26%, 31%, and 15%, respectively with short-term aerobic walking exercise.[74,75] Long-term walking programs have shown significant improvements in self-reported function (1%–11%), slowing the decline in physical function commonly seen in this disabled population (**Fig. 4**).[76–78] A randomized clinical trial of an 18-month walking program in community-dwelling older adults with knee OA reduced disability and pain, and improved balance and physical performance relative to a health education control group.[76] A biomechanical gait analysis revealed that the improved mobility of the aerobic treatment group was associated with greater knee and ankle angular velocities and vertical and anteroposterior propulsive forces,

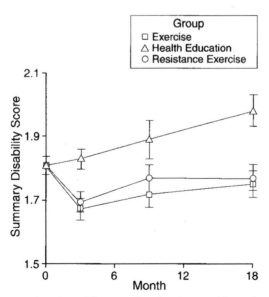

Fig. 4. Disability versus duration of intervention for the aerobic, resistance training, and health education control groups. Lower values indicate less disability. (*From* Ettinger WH Jr, Burns R, Messier SP, et al. A randomized trial comparing aerobic exercise and resistance exercise with a health education program in older adults with knee osteoarthritis. The Fitness Arthritis and Seniors Trial (FAST). JAMA 1997;277:25–31; with permission.)

characteristics that are related to faster walking speeds. In a similar cohort, higher adherence to a physical activity program was associated with better mobility and self-reported physical function.[79] The ADAPT exercise group that consisted of walking and low-intensity strength training showed statistically significant and clinically relevant (16%) long-term gains in mobility, effectively slowing the increase in mobility impairment common in an older population with OA.[43]

Aerobic exercise in older adults is more effective as a weight maintenance than a weight loss intervention. The exercise-only group in ADAPT lost 3.5 kg or 3.7% of their baseline body weight after 18 months of exercise compared with 5.2 kg and 5.7%, and 4.6 kg and 4.9% for the diet plus exercise and diet-only groups, respectively.[43] Furthermore, a 6-month aerobic exercise program resulted in a 1.8 kg weight loss, whereas the exercise and diet group lost 8.5 kg.[32] Taken together, these results indicate that long-term aerobic exercise in this disabled population improves mobility and pain, and is an effective weight maintenance intervention.

Sarcopenia and associated muscle weakness are thought to contribute to disability and pain in patients with knee OA.[80] Quadriceps weakness is an independent and modifiable risk factor for knee OA.[81,82] Muscle strengthening to combat sarcopenia and improve muscle quality in patients with knee OA is recommended in published treatment guidelines.[83,84] Over the short term (8 weeks), both low- and high-intensity strength training were effective compared with a control group; high-intensity training had more effect on knee-extensor strength (23% improvement vs 15% for low intensity).[85] Long-term low-intensity strength training in older adults with knee OA improved function, reduced pain, and improved strength relative to a health education control group.[76] In a review, Hurley and Roth[80] noted that strength training is beneficial for people with knee OA, but *the appropriate intensity and effect of long-term interventions are unclear*.

Strength training intensity or load is often defined as percent of 1 repetition maximum (%1RM).[86] High-intensity training is typically done at 70% to 85%1RM. One reason most knee OA studies use low-to-moderate regimens is a concern that the population might not tolerate intense training. King and colleagues[87] used an intensity level of 60% of baseline strength as a target resistance for patients with medial knee OA and varus alignment during a 12-week isokinetic strength-training pilot program. They defined 60%1RM as "high intensity," but the American College of Sports Medicine[86] defines it as moderate. They elicited 28% and 30% gains in knee-extensor and flexor strength at an angular velocity of 60 deg/s; however, the study lacked a control group. Knee pain did not change, and adherence was 88% across all participants. The study did show that patients with knee OA can perform strength training at higher intensity levels than previously used.

Caserotti and colleagues[88] compared changes in strength and power in old and very old healthy women assigned to either a 12-week, high-intensity (75%–80%1RM) program or a control group. The former significantly improved in strength and power relative to age-matched controls. The protocol was safe (no injuries, although 1 subject dropped out after 1 session because of "fear of injury") and well tolerated (86% completed the study). van den Ende and colleagues[89] compared 12-week, high- (70%–85% max) and low-intensity training that included dynamic weight-bearing exercises in 100 patients with rheumatoid arthritis. The high-intensity group significantly improved in strength relative to the low-intensity group with no change in measures of disease activity (medication use, swollen joint count, Ritchie index, and so forth) and an attendance rate over 75%. These studies indicate that older adult patients can tolerate high-intensity strength training, and arthritis pain is not exacerbated.

High-intensity strength training may reduce thigh fat mass and increase thigh muscle mass. An 18-week, high-intensity, lower extremity strength training program for 76- to 78-year-old healthy women significantly decreased % fat within the quadriceps (using computed tomography) versus a walking group (0.9% *decrease* for the strength training group vs a 0.7% *increase* for the walking group), and increased quadriceps lean cross-sectional area. Surprisingly, 12 weeks of high-intensity resistance training combined with a low-protein diet significantly decreased serum levels of CRP and IL-6, and this was accompanied by increased vastus lateralis muscle fiber area and increased muscle strength compared with a low-protein diet only group in older adults with chronic kidney disease.[90] A 16-week high-intensity strength training program in 20 sedentary HIV-infected men resulted in a significant decreases in total fat mass and limb fat mass (measured with dual-energy x-ray absorptiometry [DXA] scan) compared with an endurance training group.[91] Body weight decreased in both groups, with no between-group difference. In comparison with a sedentary control group, adult women who have strength trained for at least 1 year are significantly stronger, walk with a significantly lower loading rate, and have significantly fewer occurrences of heel strike transient forces, an indication of reduced loads on the lower extremity.[92] These studies indicate that short-term high-intensity strength training is well tolerated in healthy and diseased older adults, increases thigh muscle strength, decreases thigh fat depots, and reduces proinflammatory cytokines and knee joint loads. The long-term effects of this novel approach to resistance training in older adults with knee pain are untested.

EXERCISE PRESCRIPTION

Short-term and long-term aerobic and resistance training programs are safe and effective treatments for knee OA. Traditional 3 days per week, 1 hour per day programs have been the most common regimens studied. Unfortunately, little is known regarding the dose response to exercise in this older, mostly female, sedentary, and predominately overweight population. Continuous weight-bearing aerobic exercise such as walking can be difficult initially for patients with knee OA who experience significant pain. Starting with short bouts of exercise and inserting several rest periods when the patient has progressed to 30 or 40 minutes of walking will improve adherence. Adding several resistance training exercises between periods of walking has proven effective and popular with patients.[43] The intensity of the exercise intervention may differ depending on the desired outcomes. If the goal is making exercise a part of a healthy lifestyle, then continued participation is more important than intensity. The US health system remains predicated on providing acute, episodic care that is inadequate to address the altered patterns of chronic disease now facing the American public.[93] Long-term approaches that include exercise as a nonpharmacologic cotherapy should be part of the standard of care in the treatment of lower extremity OA.

SOCIAL COGNITIVE BEHAVIORAL STRATEGIES IN WEIGHT LOSS AND EXERCISE INTERVENTIONS

The reciprocal interaction of personal factors (eg, beliefs and values), social influence (eg, support and strain), and physical environment (eg, structure and access to resources) can improve weight loss and fitness by modifying both eating and physical activity behaviors.[94] We have achieved retention rates of 80% or more in 3 large-scale clinical trials (Fitness Arthritis and Seniors Trial [FAST], ADAPT, Intensive Diet and Exercise for Arthritis [IDEA]). Our protocols have evolved from social cognitive theory, group dynamics literature, and more than 15 years of clinical trials research experience.

Social cognitive theory is based on 3 constructs: self-efficacy expectations, outcome expectations, and incentives. Self-efficacy expectations represent individuals' beliefs that they can act to satisfy situational demands. Such beliefs are determined by prior behavior, physical symptoms (eg, pain, fatigue), appetite, affect, and social/environmental factors.[94] The physical activity literature has studied them in relation to the ability to perform functional tasks or physical challenges of varying difficulty,[95–97] and both the physical activity and eating behavior literatures have examined them under various environmental, social, and emotional stressors. Because self-regulation is important to successful behavior change, our clinical trials use goal setting and self-monitoring.[98,99]

Outcome expectations refer to the anticipated costs and benefits of a behavior. People are more likely to try if the perceived consequences have a favorable cost/benefit ratio.[98] Some people simply do not know the negative health effects of being overweight/obese and sedentary or are unduly optimistic about their own fate. They often become disappointed when lifestyle interventions do not meet their unrealistic expectations about how much weight they can lose, cause pain and fatigue, or prohibit a valued ethnic food.

Incentives refer to the value that people associate with outcomes.[98] In our weight-loss clinical trials, knowing how much participants value controlling their physical disability and/or reducing their weight; the dissatisfaction differential between the goal and the current weight; and the commitment to competing behaviors, such as responsibilities to families or friends, is critical information that permits the nutrition interventionist to personalize the intervention.

We train our diet and exercise interventionists in social cognitive behavioral strategies for their use with the participants. In addition, our health psychologist reviews participant progress with the interventionists biweekly and discusses strategies to use with participants who are finding it difficult to adhere to the intervention. Success stories are also discussed to reinforce successful behavioral strategies.

THE FUTURE OF WEIGHT LOSS AND EXERCISE INTERVENTIONS

The Osteoarthritis Research Society International (OARSI) guidelines recommend a combination of nonpharmacologic and pharmacologic interventions for the treatment of knee OA.[83] In addition to the challenges presented for any weight-loss intervention, the age and chronic pain associated with the knee OA population create additional barriers. Nevertheless, dietary weight-loss trials demonstrate significant improvements in pain and function with a weight loss of as little as 5%. Weight loss reduces inflammation and joint loads, but there is no evidence that disease progression is altered. A meta-analysis of previous weight loss interventions suggests that at least a 10% weight loss is necessary to have a large clinical effect.[46] Unfortunately, diet interventions lasting longer than 1 year that attain at least a 10% weight loss are rare. There are ongoing long-term efforts to determine whether a 10% weight loss has a disease-modifying effect by either slowing or stopping osteoarthritis disease progression.[68] Weight loss has beneficial effects well beyond those specific to knee OA. These include reduced risk of cardiovascular disease, type II diabetes, hypertension, foot pain, gout, and sleep apnea. Obesity is the most modifiable risk factor for knee OA and weight loss should be part of the standard of care for overweight and obese adults with knee OA.

Exercise is a safe intervention in patients with knee OA with few contraindications or adverse events. Indeed, there are few treatments that, from a public health perspective, can be delivered to a large proportion of those with OA with little associated adverse risk as exercise. Exercise therapy is recommended by all clinical guidelines for the management of knee OA and this recommendation is supported by Level 1 evidence. Previous studies have shown that standard exercise interventions for patients with knee OA (ie, walking and low-intensity strength training) result in modest improvements in pain and function without detectable effects on disease progression. Despite the strong supportive evidence, exercise is grossly underused in clinical practice.

The effectiveness of using more intense variants of exercise cotherapies to improve symptoms associated with OA, slow disease progression, and impact the underlying mechanisms of OA beyond what has been achieved with less-intense regimens is under researched; the belief being that such aggressive therapy would exacerbate OA symptoms. Indeed, the most effective combinations of intensity and duration for both aerobic and resistance interventions are unclear.

THE ROLE OF THE PHYSICIAN

The National Institutes of Health (NIH) has identified research on intervention approaches that incorporate primary care practice as a high priority.[100] Patients generally perceive that the primary care physician should have a role in weight management.[101] A recent study found that only 42% of obese adults who visited their health care professional during a 12-month span were advised to lose weight.[102] Similar results are common with physicians prescribing exercise as a primary cotherapy.[103] In visits in which either diet or exercise were discussed, a median of 0.7 minutes (42 seconds) was spent discussing the topic.[104]

Integrating the primary care physician and nurse into weight loss or exercise intervention trials has met with modest success. Ashley and colleagues[105] enrolled 113 overweight premenopausal women in a 1-year weight-loss program. A primary care office intervention (meeting with primary care physician or nurse) combined with partial meal replacements was compared with traditional dietitian-led groups with and without meal replacements. Over the course of 52 weeks, the dietitian-led group with meal replacements resulted in greater weight loss (9.1%) compared with the traditional dietitian group (4.1%) and the primary care plus meal replacement group (4.3%). All 3 groups were successful in achieving and maintaining weight loss.

A multicenter evidence-based weight management model was implemented in 47 clinical practices involving 1256 obese patients.[106] This comprehensive program involved 4 phases: setting priorities, setting guidelines, measuring performance, and improving performance. Both general practice physicians and practice nurses were recruited at each clinical site. The weight loss target was 5% to 10% of initial baseline weight. Preliminary results indicate that one-third of all patients at 12-month follow-up had a clinically relevant weight loss of greater than 5% of baseline body weight. Of the 58 general practices that began the trial, 15 dropped out primarily because of lack of resources and time. The investigators concluded that a primary care weight-management model can be used as part of a multistrategic approach to manage obesity in the community.

Primary care physicians are well positioned to have an impact on a large segment of the population with sedentary lifestyles and who are at risk for many chronic diseases.[107] Although most physicians mention physical activity to their patients, only a small percentage assess physical fitness or write a prescription for physical activity promotion programs (15%). When physicians are teamed with exercise specialists to prescribe and counsel patients to increase their physical activity, total energy expenditure, leisure time physical activity, and quality of life significantly improve in as little as 12 months.[108] The Activity Counseling Trial (ACT)[109] compared usual care physician advice with assistance (advice plus behavioral counseling at physician visits) and counseling (advice plus assistance plus regular telephone counseling and behavioral classes) and found that after 24 months, women in the assistance and counseling groups significantly increased cardiorespiratory fitness by 5%, but did not increase total physical activity. For men, there were no statistical differences between the groups in these measures. The total contact time over 24 months was 3 hours for the assistance intervention and between 5.6 (men) and 8.9 (women) hours for the counseling group. Compared with advice, the assistance intervention cost $500 per participant and the counseling cost $1100 per participant over 2 years. *Taken together, these studies suggest that involving physicians in the prescription of exercise to their patients is possible and that integrating their advice with trained exercise specialists elicits better results.*

REFERENCES

1. Fletcher E, Lewis-Faning E. Chronic rheumatic diseases: statistical study of 1000 cases of chronic rheumatism. Postgrad Med J 1945;21:137.
2. Leach RE, Baumgard S, Broom J. Obesity: its relationship to osteoarthritis of the knee. Clin Orthop 1973;93:271–3.
3. Coggon D, Reading I, Croft P, et al. Knee osteoarthritis and obesity. Int J Obes Relat Metab Disord 2001;25(5):622–7.
4. Felson DT, Zhang Y, Anthony JM, et al. Weight loss reduces the risk for symptomatic knee osteoarthritis in women. The Framingham Study. Ann Intern Med 1992;116(7):535–9.
5. Ettinger WH, Davis MA, Neuhaus JM, et al. Long-term physical functioning in persons with knee osteoarthritis from NHANES. I: effects of comorbid medical conditions. J Clin Epidemiol 1994;47(7):809–15.
6. Doherty M, Spector TD, Serni U. Session 1: epidemiology and genetics of hand osteoarthritis. Osteoarthritis Cartilage 2000;8(Suppl A):S14–5.
7. Kalichman L, Kobyliansky E. Age, body composition, and reproductive indices as predictors of radiographic hand osteoarthritis in Chuvashian women. Scand J Rheumatol 2007;36(1):53–7.
8. Davis MA, Ettinger WH, Neuhaus JM. Obesity and osteoarthritis of the knee: evidence from the National Health and Nutrition Examination Survey (NHANES I). Semin Arthritis Rheum 1990;20(3 Suppl 1):34–41.
9. Jenkins KR. Obesity's effects on the onset of functional impairment among older adults. Gerontologist 2004;44(2):206–16.
10. Ettinger WH Jr, Fried LP, Harris T, et al. Self-reported causes of physical disability in older people: the Cardiovascular Health Study. CHS Collaborative Research Group. J Am Geriatr Soc 1994;42(10):1035–44.
11. Sartorio A, Proietti M, Marinone PG, et al. Influence of gender, age and BMI on lower limb muscular power output in a large population of obese men and women. Int J Obes Relat Metab Disord 2004;28(1):91–8.
12. Miyatake N, Fujii M, Nishikawa H, et al. Clinical evaluation of muscle strength in 20-79-years-old obese Japanese. Diabetes Res Clin Pract 2000;48(1):15–21.
13. Rubenstein LZ. Falls in older people: epidemiology, risk factors and strategies for prevention. Age Ageing 2006;35(Suppl 2):ii37–41.
14. Center for Disease Control and Prevention. State-specific prevalence of obesity among adults—United States, 2005. MMWR Morb Mortal Wkly Rep 2006;55(36):985–8.

15. Kejonen P, Kauranen K, Vanharanta H. The relationship between anthropometric factors and body-balancing movements in postural balance. Arch Phys Med Rehabil 2003;84(1):17–22.
16. Jadelis K, Miller ME, Ettinger WH Jr, et al. Strength, balance, and the modifying effects of obesity and knee pain: results from the Observational Arthritis Study in Seniors (oasis). J Am Geriatr Soc 2001;49(7):884–91.
17. Riddle DL, Pulisic M, Pidcoe P, et al. Risk factors for plantar fasciitis: a matched case-control study. J Bone Joint Surg Am 2003;85(5):872–7.
18. Hills AP, Hennig EM, Byrne NM, et al. The biomechanics of adiposity—structural and functional limitations of obesity and implications for movement. Obes Rev 2002;3(1):35–43.
19. Hills AP, Hennig EM, McDonald M, et al. Plantar pressure differences between obese and non-obese adults: a biomechanical analysis. Int J Obes Relat Metab Disord 2001;25(11):1674–9.
20. Wearing SC, Hennig EM, Byrne NM, et al. Musculoskeletal disorders associated with obesity: a biomechanical perspective. Obes Rev 2006;7(3):239–50.
21. Wearing SC, Hennig EM, Byrne NM, et al. The biomechanics of restricted movement in adult obesity. Obes Rev 2006;7(1):13–24.
22. Wearing SC, Hennig EM, Byrne NM, et al. The impact of childhood obesity on musculoskeletal form. Obes Rev 2006;7(2):209–18.
23. Gravante G, Russo G, Pomara F, et al. Comparison of ground reaction forces between obese and control young adults during quiet standing on a baropodometric platform. Clin Biomech (Bristol, Avon) 2003;18(8):780–2.
24. Messier SP, Davies AB, Moore DT, et al. Severe obesity: effects on foot mechanics during walking. Foot Ankle Int 1994;15(1):29–34.
25. Chodera JD, Levell RW. Footprint patterns during walking. In: Kenedi RM, editor. Perspectives in biomedical engineering. Baltimore (MD): University Park Press; 1973. p. 81–90.
26. Liu W, Nigg BM. A mechanical model to determine the influence of masses and mass distribution on the impact force during running. J Biomech 2000;33(2):219–24.
27. Messier SP, Ettinger WH, Doyle TE, et al. Obesity: effects on gait in an osteoarthritic population. J Appl Biomech 1996;12:161–72.
28. Browning RC, Kram R. Effects of obesity on the biomechanics of walking at different speeds. Med Sci Sports Exerc 2007;39(9):1632–41.
29. Austin N, Devine A, Dick I, et al. Fear of falling in older women: a longitudinal study of incidence, persistence, and predictors. J Am Geriatr Soc 2007;55(10):1598–603.
30. Finkelstein EA, Chen H, Prabhu M, et al. The relationship between obesity and injuries among US adults. Am J Health Promot 2007;21(5):460–8.
31. DeVita P, Hortobagyi T. Obesity is not associated with increased knee joint torque and power during level walking. J Biomech 2003;36(9):1355–62.
32. Messier SP, Loeser RF, Mitchell MN, et al. Exercise and weight loss in obese older adults with knee osteoarthritis: a preliminary study. J Am Geriatr Soc 2000;48(9):1062–72.
33. Otterness IG, Swindell AC, Zimmerer RO, et al. An analysis of 14 molecular markers for monitoring osteoarthritis: segregation of the markers into clusters and distinguishing osteoarthritis at baseline. Osteoarthritis Cartilage 2000;8(3):180–5.
34. Spector TD, Hart DJ, Nandra D, et al. Low-level increases in serum C-reactive protein are present in early osteoarthritis of the knee and predict progressive disease. Arthritis Rheum 1997;40(4):723–7.

35. Van Loan MD, Johnson HL, Barbieri TF. Effect of weight loss on bone mineral content and bone mineral density in obese women. Am J Clin Nutr 1998; 67(4):734–8.
36. Goldring MB. Osteoarthritis and cartilage: the role of cytokines. Curr Rheumatol Rep 2000;2(6):459–65.
37. Sharif M, Shepstone L, Elson CJ, et al. Increased serum C reactive protein may reflect events that precede radiographic progression in osteoarthritis of the knee. Ann Rheum Dis 2000;59(1):71–4.
38. Penninx BW, Messier SP, Rejeski WJ, et al. Physical exercise and the prevention of disability in activities of daily living in older persons with osteoarthritis. Arch Intern Med 2001;161(19):2309–16.
39. Otterness IG, Weiner E, Swindell AC, et al. An analysis of 14 molecular markers for monitoring osteoarthritis. Relationship of the markers to clinical end-points. Osteoarthritis Cartilage 2001;9(3):224–31.
40. Wolfe F. The C-reactive protein but not erythrocyte sedimentation rate is associated with clinical severity in patients with osteoarthritis of the knee or hip. J Rheumatol 1997;24(8):1486–8.
41. Scharstuhl A, Glansbeek HL, van Beuningen HM, et al. Inhibition of endogenous TGF-beta during experimental osteoarthritis prevents osteophyte formation and impairs cartilage repair. J Immunol 2002;169(1):507–14.
42. Miller GD, Nicklas B, Ambrosius W, et al. Is serum leptin related to physical function and is it modifiable through weight loss and exercise in older adults with knee osteoarthritis? Int J Obes Relat Metab Disord 2004;28:1383–90.
43. Messier SP, Loeser RF, Miller GD, et al. Exercise and dietary weight loss in overweight and obese older adults with knee osteoarthritis: the Arthritis, Diet, and Activity Promotion Trial. Arthritis Rheum 2004;50(5):1501–10.
44. Miller GD, Nicklas BJ, Davis C, et al. Intensive weight loss program improves physical function in older obese adults with knee osteoarthritis. Obesity (Silver Spring) 2006;14(7):1219–30.
45. Christensen R, Astrup A, Bliddal H. Weight loss: the treatment of choice for knee osteoarthritis? A randomized trial. Osteoarthritis Cartilage 2005;13(1):20–7.
46. Christensen R, Bartels EM, Astrup A, et al. Effect of weight reduction in obese patients diagnosed with knee osteoarthritis: a systematic review and meta-analysis. Ann Rheum Dis 2007;66(4):433–9.
47. Wedick NM, Barrett-Connor E, Knoke JD, et al. The relationship between weight loss and all-cause mortality in older men and women with and without diabetes mellitus: the Rancho Bernardo study. J Am Geriatr Soc 2002;50(11):1810–5.
48. Newman AB, Yanez D, Harris T, et al. Weight change in old age and its association with mortality. J Am Geriatr Soc 2001;49(10):1309–18.
49. Shea MK, Houston DK, Nicklas BJ, et al. The effect of randomization to weight loss on total mortality in older overweight and obese adults: the ADAPT Study. J Gerontol A Biol Sci Med Sci 2010;65(5):519–25.
50. Diehr P, Newman AB, Jackson SA, et al. Weight-modification trials in older adults: what should the outcome measure be? Curr Control Trials Cardiovasc Med 2002;3(1):1.
51. Andersen RE, Wadden TA, Herzog RJ. Changes in bone mineral content in obese dieting women. Metabolism 1997;46(8):857–61.
52. Hyldstrup L, Andersen T, McNair P, et al. Bone metabolism in obesity: changes related to severe overweight and dietary weight reduction. Acta Endocrinol (Copenh) 1993;129(5):393–8.

53. Andersen RE, Wadden TA, Bartlett SJ, et al. Relation of weight loss to changes in serum lipids and lipoproteins in obese women. Am J Clin Nutr 1995;62:350–7.

54. Ensrud KE, Cauley J, Lipschutz R, et al. Weight change and fractures in older women. Study of Osteoporotic Fractures Research Group. Arch Intern Med 1997;157(8):857–63.

55. Fiatarone Singh MA. Combined exercise and dietary intervention to optimize body composition in aging. Ann N Y Acad Sci 1998;854:378–93.

56. Janssen I, Fortier A, Hudson R, et al. Effects of an energy-restrictive diet with or without exercise on abdominal fat, intermuscular fat, and metabolic risk factors in obese women. Diabetes Care 2002;25(3):431–8.

57. Wang X, Miller GD, Messier SP, et al. Knee strength maintained despite loss of lean body mass during weight loss in older obese adults with knee osteoarthritis. J Gerontol A Biol Sci Med Sci 2007;62(8):866–71.

58. Wadden TA, Vogt RA, Andersen RE, et al. Exercise in the treatment of obesity: effects of four interventions on body composition, resting energy expenditure, appetite, and mood. J Consult Clin Psychol 1997;65(2):269–77.

59. Wadden TA, Berkowitz RI, Sarwer DB, et al. Benefits of lifestyle modification in the pharmacologic treatment of obesity: a randomized trial. Arch Intern Med 2001;161(2):218–27.

60. Kayman S, Bruvold W, Stern JS. Maintenance and relapse after weight loss in women: behavioral aspects. Am J Clin Nutr 1990;52(5):800–7.

61. Perri MG, Martin AD, Leermakers EA, et al. Effects of group- versus home-based exercise in the treatment of obesity. J Consult Clin Psychol 1997;65(2):278–85.

62. Wing RR, Epstein LH, Paternostro-Bayles M, et al. Exercise in a behavioural weight control programme for obese patients with type 2 (non-insulin-dependent) diabetes. Diabetologia 1988;31(12):902–9.

63. Perri MG, McAllister DA, Gange JJ, et al. Effects of four maintenance programs on the long-term management of obesity. J Consult Clin Psychol 1988;56(4):529–34.

64. Esposito K, Pontillo A, Di Palo C, et al. Effect of weight loss and lifestyle changes on vascular inflammatory markers in obese women: a randomized trial. JAMA 2003;289(14):1799–804.

65. Pirozzo S, Summerbell C, Cameron C, et al. Advice on low-fat diets for obesity. Cochrane Database Syst Rev 2002;(2):CD003640.

66. Bravata DM, Sanders L, Huang J, et al. Efficacy and safety of low-carbohydrate diets: a systematic review. JAMA 2003;289(14):1837–50.

67. Heymsfield SB, van Mierlo CA, van der Knaap HC, et al. Weight management using a meal replacement strategy: meta and pooling analysis from six studies. Int J Obes Relat Metab Disord 2003;27(5):537–49.

68. Messier SP, Legault C, Mihalko S, et al. The Intensive Diet and Exercise for Arthritis (IDEA) trial: design and rationale. BMC Musculoskelet Disord 2009; 10:93.

69. Roddy E, Zhang W, Doherty M. Aerobic walking or strengthening exercise for osteoarthritis of the knee? A systematic review. Ann Rheum Dis 2005;64(4):544–8.

70. Patrick DL, Ramsey SD, Spencer AC, et al. Economic evaluation of aquatic exercise for persons with osteoarthritis. Med Care 2001;39(5):413–24.

71. Wyatt FB, Milam S, Manske RC, et al. The effects of aquatic and traditional exercise programs on persons with knee osteoarthritis. J Strength Cond Res 2001; 15(3):337–40.

72. Suomi R. Effectiveness of Arthritis Foundation aquatic program on strength and range of motion in women with arthritis. J Aging Phys Act 1997;5:341–51.
73. Suomi R, Collier D. Effects of arthritis exercise programs on functional fitness and perceived activities of daily living measures in older adults with arthritis. Arch Phys Med Rehabil 2003;84(11):1589–94.
74. Minor MA, Hewett JE, Webel RR, et al. Efficacy of physical conditioning exercise in patients with rheumatoid arthritis and osteoarthritis. Arthritis Rheum 1989; 32(11):1396–405.
75. Kovar PA, Allegrante JP, MacKenzie CR, et al. Supervised fitness walking in patients with osteoarthritis of the knee. A randomized, controlled trial. Ann Intern Med 1992;116(7):529–34.
76. Ettinger WH Jr, Burns R, Messier SP, et al. A randomized trial comparing aerobic exercise and resistance exercise with a health education program in older adults with knee osteoarthritis. The Fitness Arthritis and Seniors Trial (FAST). JAMA 1997;277(1):25–31.
77. Thomas KS, Muir KR, Doherty M, et al. Home based exercise programme for knee pain and knee osteoarthritis: randomised controlled trial. BMJ 2002; 325(7367):752.
78. van Baar ME, Assendelft WJ, Dekker J, et al. Effectiveness of exercise therapy in patients with osteoarthritis of the hip or knee: a systematic review of randomized clinical trials. Arthritis Rheum 1999;42(7):1361–9.
79. van Gool CH, Penninx BWJH, Kempen GIJM, et al. Effects of exercise adherence on osteoarthritis-related performance and disability. Arthritis Care Res 2005;53(1):24–32.
80. Hurley BF, Roth SM. Strength training in the elderly: effects on risk factors for age-related diseases. Sports Med 2000;30(4):249–68.
81. Hootman JM, Fitzgerald SJ, Macera CA, et al. Lower extremity muscle strength and risk of self-reported hip or knee osteoarthritis. J Phys Act Health 2004;1(4):321–30.
82. Slemenda C, Brandt KD, Heilman DK, et al. Quadriceps weakness and osteoarthritis of the knee. Ann Intern Med 1997;127(2):97–104.
83. Zhang W, Moskowitz RW, Nuki G, et al. OARSI recommendations for the management of hip and knee osteoarthritis, Part II: OARSI evidence-based, expert consensus guidelines. Osteoarthritis Cartilage 2008;16(2):137–62.
84. American Academy of Orthopaedic Surgeons. Treatment of osteoarthritis of the knee (non-arthroplasty). J Am Acad Orthop Surg 2008:19–20. Available at: http://www.aaos.org/Research/guidelines/GuidelineOAKnee.asp. Accessed May 17, 2010.
85. Jan MH, Lin JJ, Liau JJ, et al. Investigation of clinical effects of high- and low-resistance training for patients with knee osteoarthritis: a randomized controlled trial. Phys Ther 2008;88(4):427–36.
86. Kraemer WJ, Adams K, Cafarelli E, et al. Progression models in resistance training for healthy adults. Med Sci Sports Exerc 2002;34(2):364–80.
87. King LK, Birmingham TB, Kean CO, et al. Resistance training for medial compartment knee osteoarthritis and malalignment. Med Sci Sports Exerc 2008;40(8):1376–84.
88. Caserotti P, Aagaard P, Larsen JB, et al. Explosive heavy-resistance training in old and very old adults: changes in rapid muscle force, strength and power. Scand J Med Sci Sports 2008;18(6):773–82.
89. van den Ende CH, Hazes JM, le CS, et al. Comparison of high and low intensity training in well controlled rheumatoid arthritis. Results of a randomised clinical trial. Ann Rheum Dis 1996;55(11):798–805.

90. Castaneda C, Gordon PL, Parker RC, et al. Resistance training to reduce the malnutrition-inflammation complex syndrome of chronic kidney disease. Am J Kidney Dis 2004;43(4):607–16.

91. Lindegaard B, Hansen T, Hvid T, et al. The effect of strength and endurance training on insulin sensitivity and fat distribution in HIV-infected patients with lipodystrophy. J Clin Endocrinol Metab 2008;93(10):3860–9.

92. Mikesky AE, Meyer A, Thompson KL. Relationship between quadriceps strength and rate of loading during gait in women. J Orthop Res 2000;18(2):171–5.

93. Thorpe KE, Ogden LL, Galactionova K. Chronic conditions account for rise in Medicare spending from 1987 to 2006. Health Aff (Millwood) 2010;29(4):718–24.

94. Bandura A. Self-efficacy: the exercise of control. New York: W H Freeman and Co; 1997.

95. McAuley E, Blissmer B. Self-efficacy determinants and consequences of physical activity. Exerc Sport Sci Rev 2000;28(2):85–8.

96. McAuley E, Blissmer B, Katula J, et al. Physical activity, self-esteem, and self-efficacy relationships in older adults: a randomized controlled trial. Ann Behav Med 2000;22(2):131–9.

97. McAuley E, Blissmer B, Katula J, et al. Exercise environment, self-efficacy, and affective responses to acute exercise in older adults. Psychol Health 2000;15(3):341–55.

98. McAuley E, Mihalko SL. Measuring exercise-related self-efficacy. In: Duda JL, editor. Advances in sport and exercise psychology measurement. Morgantown (WV): Fitness Information Technology, Inc; 1998. p. 371–89.

99. Rejeski WJ, Mihalko SL. Physical activity and quality of life in older adults. J Gerontol A Biol Sci Med Sci 2001;56:23–35.

100. Blair SN, Applegate WB, Dunn AL, et al. Activity Counseling Trial (ACT): rationale, design, and methods. Activity Counseling Trial Research Group. Med Sci Sports Exerc 1998;30(7):1097–106.

101. Tan D, Zwar NA, Dennis SM, et al. Weight management in general practice: what do patients want? Med J Aust 2006;185(2):73–5.

102. Galuska DA, Will JC, Serdula MK, et al. Are health care professionals advising obese patients to lose weight? JAMA 1999;282(16):1576–8.

103. Bennell KL, Hunt MA, Wrigley TV, et al. Muscle and exercise in the prevention and management of knee osteoarthritis: an internal medicine specialist's guide. Med Clin North Am 2009;93(1):161–77, xii.

104. Flocke SA, Stange KC. Direct observation and patient recall of health behavior advice. Prev Med 2004;38(3):343–9.

105. Ashley JM, St Jeor ST, Schrage JP, et al. Weight control in the physician's office. Arch Intern Med 2001;161(13):1599–604.

106. The Counterweight Project Team. A new evidence-based model for weight management in primary care: the counterweight programme. J Hum Nutr Diet 2004;17:191–208.

107. Petrella RJ, Lattanzio CN, Overend TJ. Physical activity counseling and prescription among Canadian primary care physicians. Arch Intern Med 2007;167(16):1774–81.

108. Elley CR, Kerse N, Arroll B, et al. Effectiveness of counselling patients on physical activity in general practice: cluster randomised controlled trial. BMJ 2003;326(7393):793.

109. Writing Group for the Activity Counseling Trial Research Group. Effects of physical activity counseling in primary care: the Activity Counseling Trial: a randomized controlled trial. JAMA 2001;286(6):677–87.

Device Use: Walking Aids, Braces, and Orthoses for Symptomatic Knee Osteoarthritis

K. Douglas Gross, PT, ScD

KEYWORDS

• Walking aids • Orthoses • Knee • Osteoarthritis

Osteoarthritis (OA) is a growing epidemic, and there is no known cure for the condition. In 2005, there were 27 million Americans with physician-diagnosed OA.[1] By 2020, that number will have doubled,[2] largely because of the rapid aging of the general population and soaring rates of obesity. When OA becomes symptomatic in the knee, as it does in at least 1 out of every 8 adults more than 60 years of age,[3,4] the effect can be debilitating. Mobility limitations account for 80% of all chronic disabilities among seniors,[5] and knee OA is the single most prevalent cause.[6]

Despite increasing concern about the capacity of our health care system to respond to this rising demand, routine care for knee OA has changed little in several decades. A visit to the family doctor rarely results in more than a prescription for palliative drugs and the promise of watchful waiting. Few attempts are made to identify interventions capable of supporting the structural integrity of an osteoarthritic knee, or to help restore its capacity to bear weight, sustain loads, and perform the functions that allow continued participation in activities. Instead, this progressive disease is allowed to persist, and narrowly focused treatments target only short-term symptom reduction using palliative drugs. The 2 most widely prescribed drugs, the nonsteroidal antiinflammatory drugs (NSAIDs) and cyclooxygenase-2 (COX-2) inhibitors have recently come under intense public scrutiny for their alarmingly high rate of adverse events[7,8] and their grossly immoderate cost.[9] With no physical protection from further damage, knee OA tends to worsen with time. Eventually the patient's activity limitations become severe enough to necessitate surgical joint replacement. If this pattern of medical practice continues, the number of primary total knee athroplasties performed each year in the United States will increase 632% between 2004 and 2030, reaching an estimated 3.5 million annually.[4]

Graduate Programs in Physical Therapy, MGH Institute of Health Professions, Charlestown Navy Yard, 36 First Avenue, Boston, MA 02129-4557, USA
E-mail address: kdgross@mghihp.edu

Clin Geriatr Med 26 (2010) 479–502
doi:10.1016/j.cger.2010.03.007
0749-0690/10/$ – see front matter © 2010 Elsevier Inc. All rights reserved.

With few conservative options available in the medical system, increasing numbers of OA sufferers are turning to untested folk remedies and self-prescribed dietary supplements. There is enormous popular demand for noninvasive and nonpharmacologic therapies for OA, and there is a pressing need for physicians to respond to this demand by updating their patterns of practice. The following narrative review introduces physicians to several of the most important noninvasive devices used in the conservative management of symptomatic knee OA. Each section of the review opens with a presentation of the device's anticipated biomechanical effects and then considers evidence of clinical efficacy. Where possible, summary comments are offered that communicate the author's subjective experience prescribing these devices, and some considerations that have been found to be important for successful patient management are also discussed.

TARGETING KNEE BIOMECHANICS

The knee consists of 3 distinct joint compartments: the medial tibiofemoral (TF), the lateral TF, and the patellofemoral (PF). The shared goal of many noninvasive devices for knee OA is to alter lower limb biomechanics to limit the exposure of 1 or more of these knee compartments to potentially damaging and provocative mechanical stresses. Optimal prescription of a device requires that physicians specify not only the knee compartments requiring protection but also the types of mechanical stress that should be reduced within these compartments. A basic understanding of lower limb biomechanics can valuably inform this determination.

WALKING AIDS AND GROUND REACTION FORCES

Nearly all patients with symptomatic knee OA report symptom provocation with some type of weight-bearing activity, which indicates that sensitivity to mechanical load is a common feature of the most frequently symptomatic knee compartments. Physicians charged with caring for patients with medial or lateral TF OA are familiar with the symptomatic and functional improvements that often occur when patients are provided with assistive walking devices that reduce compressive loading over TF joint surfaces.[10,11]

When body weight is borne on a limb during standing (**Fig. 1**) or walking (**Fig. 2**), the limb is subjected to an equal and opposite reaction force from the ground. The vertical component of this ground reaction force (GRF) exerts a compressive load on the weight-bearing surfaces of the TF joint. In bilateral standing, the GRF loads each limb with approximately 50% of body weight. By contrast, the unilateral stance phase of self-paced walking generates a peak GRF equal to 150% to 200% body weight. For knees with symptomatic medial or lateral TF OA, this amount of compressive load can soon become excessive. When a walker, cane, crutch, or similar assistive walking device is used, a portion of body weight can be shifted off the symptomatic limb and onto the partial weight-bearing device. The shifting of body weight off a symptomatic limb results in a proportionate reduction in the GRF acting on that limb, and a consequent lessening of the compressive load that is exerted on symptomatic TF compartments.[12] It is by means of this reduction in the compressive load on symptomatic TF joint compartments that walkers and canes are so often effective in improving tolerance for upright activities among seniors with knee OA. Shopping is an example of an upright activity for which walker or cane use may be indicated. Shopping can involve long periods of uninterrupted standing and walking, and shopping is typically one of the first activity limitations reported by older women with medial or lateral TF OA.

STANDING
Anterior view

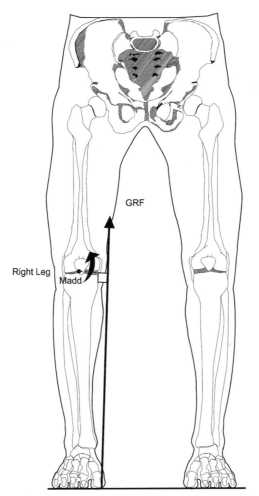

Fig. 1. Ground reaction force (GRF) through a normally aligned knee during standing. The perpendicular distance of the GRF from the knee's axis of rotation produces an adduction moment (M_{add}) that concentrates compressive load on the medial TF compartment.

CANES AND THE ADDUCTION MOMENT

In addition to the widespread benefits afforded to medial and lateral TF compartments by an assistive walking device that reduces the overall magnitude of the GRF, there is also a second way in which a unilaterally held assistive walking device (such as a cane or walking stick) can be made particularly effective in reducing compressive load more specifically on a symptomatic medial TF compartment. This second mechanism depends on the cane's placement relative to the knee's axis of frontal plane rotation (located near the center of the knee). However, to take meaningful advantage of this second mechanism, a cane or walking stick must be held in the hand contralateral

Walking
Anterior view

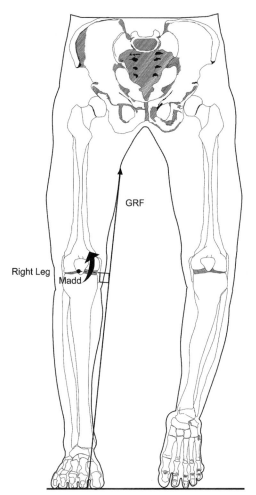

Fig. 2. GRF through a normally aligned knee during walking. Although the magnitude of the GRF is only 50% of body weight during standing, it may be 150% to 200% of body weight during walking. The perpendicular distance of the GRF from the knee's axis of rotation produces an adduction moment (M_{add}) that concentrates compressive load on the medial TF compartment.

to the symptomatic knee so that it can be made to contact the ground at some distance from the symptomatic medial TF compartment.

During standing, the GRF normally passes a short distance medial to the knee's axis of frontal plane rotation (see **Fig. 1**). As a result of the short distance over which it is applied, the GRF generates a small torque, or adduction moment (M_{add}), that attempts to rotate the tibia around the knee's axis of frontal plane motion in the direction of knee adduction. The additional adduction stress on the knee serves to concentrate compressive load on the medial TF compartment. Although the extra compressive load may be tolerable during quiet standing, the heightened stresses of walking can quickly overwhelm a knee with symptomatic medial TF OA. Not only is the GRF of a greater magnitude in walking than in standing, its vector is also a greater distance medial of the knee (see **Fig. 2**). At its peak in the early stance phase, the resulting adduction moment causes the medial TF compartment to absorb at least 60% to 70% of the knee's total compressive load.[13] Given the magnitude of compressive load to which the medial TF compartment is repeatedly exposed during walking, it is advisable for many patients with symptomatic medial TF OA to use a cane held in the contralateral hand whenever they are ambulating for long periods.

The downward force that a patient applies to the cane generates its own equal and opposite GRF at the point where the cane contacts the ground. This GRF (labeled GRF_{cane} in **Fig. 3**) acts through the contralateral upper extremity and trunk to generate a moment of force at the symptomatic knee (labeled M_{cane} in **Fig. 3**) which counteracts the usual M_{add}. By having the cane make ground contact at some distance contralateral to the symptomatic knee, the patient is able to take useful advantage of a long lever arm over which to apply this protective abductory moment of force. More importantly, by effectively resisting the forces that drive the knee into greater adduction, the patient succeeds in protecting the medial TF compartment against potentially

Cane Use
Anterior view

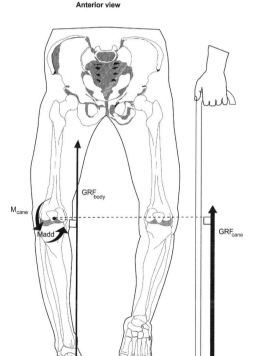

Fig. 3. Partial weight bearing on a cane also generates a GRF (GRF_{cane}). When the cane is held in the hand contralateral to the symptomatic knee, the GRF_{cane} is applied over a long lever arm to generate a moment of force (M_{cane}) that counteracts the usual adduction moment (M_{add}) at the knee. In so doing, contralateral cane use is effective in reducing load over the medial TF compartment.

damaging levels of compressive load.[12] However, to make use of a cane for this purpose, proper sizing and placement are critical.

To properly fit a cane to a patient, the cane should be aligned alongside the contra-lateral leg and contacting the ground just lateral of the lateral malleolus. The height of the cane is then adjusted until the handle is approximately level with the superior tip of the greater trochanter (**Fig. 4**). The user's arm should maintain 20 to 30 degrees of elbow flexion while holding the cane in this position. To successfully bolster against the effects of the M_{add} when it reaches its peak magnitude during walking, the patient must initiate partial weight bearing through the cane at the same instant that the foot of the affected limb strikes the ground (ie, at the onset of stance phase). Guided rehearsal of the correct walking pattern is often necessary, especially for older patients.

Cane Sizing
Anterior view

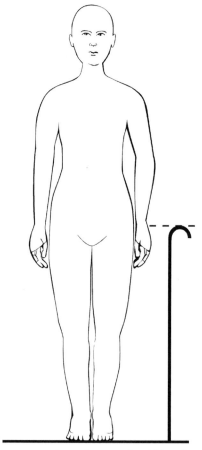

Fig. 4. To properly fit a cane to a patient, the cane should be aligned alongside the leg and contacting the ground just lateral of the lateral malleolus. The height of the cane is then adjusted until the handle is approximately level with the superior tip of the greater trochanter.

The author is not aware of any trials that have specifically evaluated the clinical efficacy of cane use. However, the American College of Rheumatology (ACR)[14] and the European League Against Rheumatism (EULAR)[15] recommend cane prescription as an important component of conservative medical care for knee and hip OA. A cane used in the contralateral hand has been shown to reduce intraarticular loading at the hip joint by 50% during self-paced walking,[16] and reductions in the knee M_{add} of more than 10% have been reported among patients with medial TF OA.[12] Because the PF compartment is not directly exposed to large weight-bearing loads during most upright standing or level-ground walking activities, cane use is not expected to serve any essential purpose for patients whose symptoms are of strictly PF origin.

THE UNLOADER BRACE AND GENU VARUM/VALGUM MALALIGNMENT

Although the magnitude and direction of the GRF determines how much overall compressive load the TF joint routinely sustains, the relative bony alignment of the tibia and femur also has an enormous effect on the manner in which this compressive load is distributed across the medial and lateral compartments. As little as 5 degrees of genu varum (bowlegged) malalignment results in an estimated 70% to 90% increase in compressive load over the medial TF compartment (**Fig. 5**).[17] This dramatic increase in compressive loading medially corresponds to a fourfold increase in the odds of OA worsening in the medial TF compartment over 18 months.[18] Conversely, genu valgum (knock-kneed) malalignment increases compressive load on the lateral TF compartment and increases the chance of worsening lateral TF OA fivefold in the same period.[18]

Relevant genu varum or valgum malalignments are often identifiable during simple visual inspection of a patient's relaxed standing posture. Busy physicians should be reassured to know that simple clinical measurements of TF alignment (using a hand-held goniometer) correlate well with the more cumbersome measurements taken from long-limb radiographs.[19] When genu varum malalignment is accompanied by knee instability, as is often the case with more severe medial TF OA, the bowlegged posture of the limb may become visibly exaggerated under the influence of the large M_{add} that occurs during walking. In such instances, observation of the patient's walking pattern will reveal an abrupt thrust of the knee into an exaggerated varus (bowlegged) attitude with each successive footfall. Among knees with moderate genu varum malalignment in standing, the additional presence of an observable varus thrust during walking has been found to increase the odds of medial TF OA progression threefold in 18-months.[20]

Improved frontal-plane knee alignment and mediolateral stability against thrust are commonly cited reasons for prescribing a valgus-inducing unloader brace to patients with medial TF OA, or (less commonly) a varus-inducing unloader brace to patients with lateral TF OA.[21] However, nearly all attempts to realign a knee in a way that reduces compressive load on the medial TF compartment are likely to simultaneously result in increased compressive load on the lateral TF compartment. The converse is also true. Thus, in most cases, prescription of an unloader brace should be reserved for patients with at least moderate genu varum or valgum malalignment, and symptomatic TF OA that is primarily unicompartmental.

When a realigning force is applied to the knee using a valgus-inducing unloader brace for medial TF OA (**Fig. 6**), the expectation is that slight improvements in TF alignment and stability (ie, reduced genu varum malalignment and reduced varus knee thrust) will result in meaningful reductions in the magnitude of the M_{add}, and consequent improvement in the distribution of compressive load over TF joint surfaces.

Genu Varum Malalignment
Anterior View in Walking

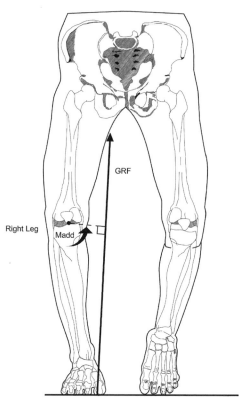

Fig. 5. Loading of the knee with genu varum, or bowlegged, malalignment. Genu varum increases the adduction moment (M_{add}) at the knee and the magnitude of compressive load on the medial TF compartment.

Using video fluoroscopy, Komistek and colleagues[22] confirmed that a custom-fitted unloader brace is capable of producing desirable changes in TF alignment that are maintained during walking. Among 15 men and women with unicompartmental OA in the medial or lateral TF joint, only the 3 most obese subjects failed to maintain the expected improvements in joint alignment during treadmill ambulation. The mean change in TF alignment was 2.2 degrees, which corresponded to a mean increase in joint space of 1.2 mm in the targeted TF compartment. These desirable changes help to explain the 10% to 13% reductions in the M_{add} that other investigators have reported in association with valgus-inducing unloader braces.[23,24] As the braced knee assumes a more erect alignment, the distance between the knee's axis of rotation and the GRF is reduced, causing the M_{add} to lessen and compressive load to become more evenly distributed over the medial and lateral TF compartments.

Although the mechanical effects of a properly fitted unloader brace can be safely inferred from gait laboratory investigations, few high-quality clinical trials are available to help inform an assessment of the likely clinical effects of an unloader brace. A 2008 update of a 2005 Cochrane review[25] succeeded in identifying only 2 trials that were of sufficient quality to satisfy all criteria for inclusion. In one, Kirkley and colleagues[26] compared the mean change in measured pain and function following 6 months of a prescribed valgus-inducing unloader brace (n = 41) with the effects of no brace (n = 33), or a neoprene sleeve (n = 36). All subjects had medial TF OA with genu varum malalignment in standing (mean 9 degrees genu varum). The prescribed Generation II unloader brace (Generation II Orthotics, Richmond, British Columbia, Canada) was custom fitted, and consisted of lightweight calf and thigh shells connected on the medial side by an adjustable hinge (see **Fig. 6**). Tension in the brace was adjusted to apply as much as 4 degrees valgus correction.

Results of the trial by Kirkley and colleagues[26] indicated that the group receiving the valgus-inducing unloader brace achieved greater mean improvements in pain and function after 6 months than either of the 2 comparison groups. The mean change score for pain (lowest score possible was −500 mm) was −13.1 mm for the control group, 13.1 mm for the neoprene sleeve group, and 43.2 mm for the unloader brace group ($P = .001$). The mean change score for physical function (lowest score possible was −1700 mm) was −6.5 mm for the control group, 68.9 mm for the neoprene sleeve group, and 157.2 mm for the unloader brace group ($P = .004$).

The second trial, a multicenter randomized controlled trial by Brouwer and colleagues,[27] enrolled 117 subjects with unicompartmental OA in the medial or lateral TF compartments and genu varum or valgum malalignment in standing. The prescribed unloader braces in this trial consisted of calf and thigh shells in 4 generic sizes that were connected by heavy metal hinges on the medial and lateral sides. The hinges allowed for adjustment of up to 12.5 degrees valgus correction for subjects with medial TF OA, and up to 10 degrees varus correction for subjects with lateral TF OA. At 12 months, an intent-to-treat comparison of 60 subjects assigned to the treatment group (including those with varus-inducing or valgus-inducing knee braces) and

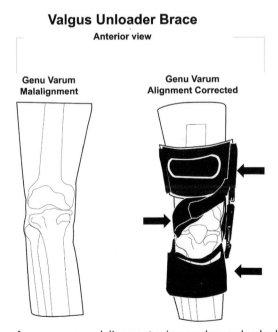

Valgus Unloader Brace

Anterior view

Genu Varum Malalignment   **Genu Varum Alignment Corrected**

Fig. 6. Correction of genu varum malalignment using a valgus unloader brace.

57 subjects in the unbraced control group revealed only nonsignificant differences with respect to overall pain reduction. However, brace users also reported a mean increase in walking tolerance that was 1.8 km greater than the increase reported by controls ($P = .04$). A functional treatment effect of this magnitude is likely to be of substantial benefit to patients experiencing difficulty walking long distances because of unicompartmental TF OA.

Before recommending an unloader brace to a patient with unicompartmental TF OA, it should be noted that, of the 60 subjects originally assigned to intervention in the trial by Brouwer and colleagues,[27] more than one-third (n = 24) stopped using the generically sized brace before completion of the 12-month treatment period. The most commonly cited reasons for nonadherence were a lack of noticeable benefit (n = 20) and poor fit (n = 4). This report reinforces the author's own clinical experience. Obese patients have particular trouble with generically sized unloader braces, and older women commonly express frustration with the bulkiness and inconvenience of many metal-hinged braces. Younger and slimmer patients are easier to fit with an unloader brace, but some customization is often necessary to ensure that the desired mechanical effects are retained. There is increasing evidence that the mediolateral stability offered by a snugly fitting custom brace may be critical to ensuring that the desired reductions in mechanical stress are achieved.[21] To date, there have been no clinical trials evaluating the specific effects of an unloader brace among older adults with an observable varus thrust, although it seems reasonable to suppose that a snugly fitting unloader brace might be of special benefit to these patients.

A challenge faced by prescribing physicians is how best to match a particular unloader brace with a particular patient's needs and preferences. Consultation with a knowledgeable physical therapist or orthotist may be helpful. In the interest of improving patient adherence, it is best to specify that the patient use the brace only during particular aggravating activities. Adherence is more likely when the brace is used successfully to improve tolerance for recreational walking, shopping, tennis, or some other weight-bearing pastime.

PATELLAR TAPING OR BRACING AND RETROPATELLAR PRESSURE

It has been assumed that knee OA was less common in the PF than in the TF compartments. It now seems that this assumption was incorrect.[28] Among subjects reporting knee symptoms in the Framingham Study, 40% had radiographic OA that remained isolated to 1 or both of the TF compartments, whereas 60% exhibited OA that was isolated to (20%) or inclusive of (40%) the PF compartment.[29] PF joint involvement is even more common among women,[30] and, because pathologic changes at the PF joint less frequently exhibit early osteophytosis, OA in the PF compartment probably goes undiagnosed far more often than OA elsewhere in the knee.[31] When radiographic OA is identified in the PF compartment, the changes there often provide a better explanation for the activity limitations that a person experiences than do osteoarthritic changes in either of the TF compartments.[30]

Because it is now known that involvement of the PF compartment is common among older people with knee pain, it is surprising that so few trials have been undertaken to evaluate the efficacy of patellar taping and bracing interventions for persons with PF OA. Instead, most of what is currently known about PF devices has been abstracted from previous studies of their use among young adults with PF pain syndrome. Studied application of these interventions to older patients with knee OA is an overdue arrival, and how the design of these devices might be modified to maximize their usefulness in older populations is poorly understood.

The knee typically flexes less than 15 degrees during the weight-bearing phase of level-ground walking.[32] As a result, the patella rarely engages the femur during many upright activities. In contrast, the actions of climbing a stair and rising from a chair require maximum joint angles of more than 90 degrees.[33,34] During these activities, with the GRF passing a substantial distance posterior of the knee's axis of sagittal plane rotation, the quadriceps muscle must contract powerfully to counteract a sizable external moment of force for knee flexion (**Fig. 7**). When ascending stairs, the peak external knee flexion moment rises to 4 times the magnitude of the peak M_{add} during the same effort.[35] The required quadriceps contraction exerts enormous compressive load on the PF joint. Load on PF joint is equivalent to 3 to 4 times body weight during unassisted stair climbing, and may be as much as 7 to 8 times body weight when rising from a low chair.[36]

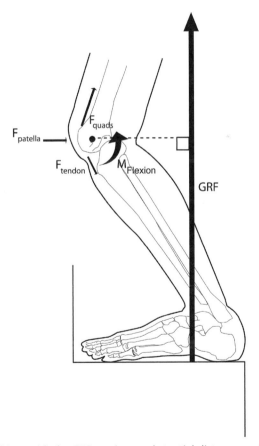

Stair Climbing
Lateral view

Fig. 7. In stair climbing, with the GRF passing a substantial distance posterior of the knee's axis of rotation, the quadriceps muscle must contract powerfully (F_{quads}) to counteract a sizable external moment of force for knee flexion ($M_{flexion}$). The contraction increases compressive load at the PF joint ($F_{patella}$).

Despite the enormous compressive stress that is exerted on the PF joint during weight-bearing knee flexion, clinical experience indicates that knee flexion in a closed kinematic chain (foot planted on a stationary ground) is typically better tolerated than similarly resisted knee flexion in an open kinematic chain (foot free to move). This apparent inconsistency is explained by the retropatellar contact area being markedly increased during closed-chain knee function.[37] The increased contact area means that the overall compressive load on the PF joint can be distributed over a greater surface area. With a greater surface area over which to distribute the compressive load, retropatellar pressure (pressure = compressive load/contact area) on the articular surfaces of the PF joint is reduced (**Fig. 8**).

PF taping and bracing interventions seek to reduce retropatellar pressure by maximizing PF contact area during weight-bearing activities involving knee flexion. These treatments are believed to be ideal in cases in which pressure on the lateral PF joint surfaces is made excessive by lateral patellar malalignment or lateral PF instability. However, contrary to theory, the benefits of patellar taping and bracing may not be entirely specific to patients with either of these clinical findings. One recently derived clinical prediction rule[38] suggests that the likelihood of a younger patient with PF pain responding to medially directed patellar taping (**Fig. 9**) increases when there is sufficient suppleness and flexibility in the lateral patellar soft tissues. This suggestion is contrary to the usual notion that tightness in the lateral soft tissues is a primary cause of the lateral patellar malalignment that indicates the need for realigning interventions. Moreover, there is little evidence supporting the claim that the usual methods of applying tape succeed in maintaining a measurable medial displacement of the patella once weight-bearing knee flexion activity has been initiated.[39,40] A far more consistent effect of patellar taping and bracing interventions is to increase contact area between the medial and lateral load-bearing facets of the patella and the underlying medial and lateral trochlea of the femur. For example, Powers and colleagues[41] used dynamic magnetic resonance imaging (MRI) to image PF contact at 4 different angles of weight-bearing knee flexion. Among the 15 symptomatic female participants, both of the patellar braces evaluated (the On-Track [Don Joy Inc., Vista, California] and the Patellar Tracking Orthosis [Breg Inc., Vista, California]) were effective in increasing mean PF contact area by 20% to 25% in comparison with the no-brace condition.

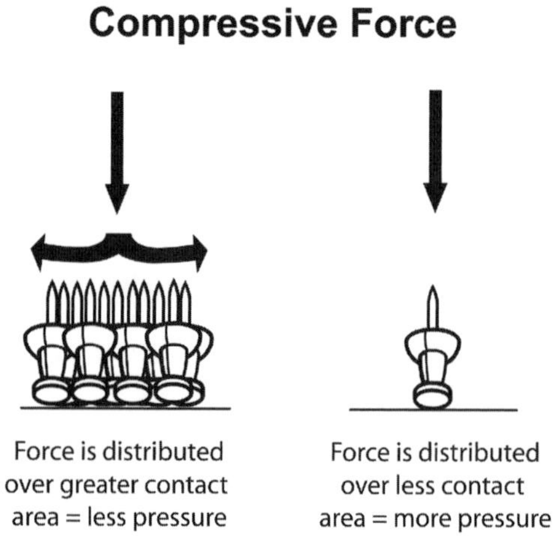

Compressive Force

Force is distributed
over greater contact
area = less pressure

Force is distributed
over less contact
area = more pressure

Fig. 8. Focal compressive stress is measured as pressure. Because pressure is equal to the compressive force per unit of contact area, pressure declines when contact area is increased.

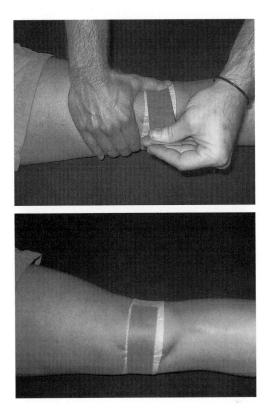

Fig. 9. Medially directed patellar taping increases PF contact area so that retropatellar pressure is reduced.

This sizable increase in PF contact area was concurrent with a mean reduction in knee pain of 45% to 50%. Neither lateral patellar malalignment nor lateral patellar instability was a prerequisite for participation in the study.

A recent systematic review and meta-analysis[42] synthesized the current best evidence relating to the clinical effects of patellar taping and bracing for the treatment of chronic knee pain in older and younger adults. Of the 16 studies that satisfied the criteria for inclusion, 13 investigated taping or bracing effects in nonspecific anterior knee pain, whereas only 3 studies evaluated the effects of patellar taping among subjects with diagnosed knee OA. Of these 3 studies, none required that participants exhibit any radiographic or clinical confirmation of PF compartment involvement. Consequently, the results of these trials must be interpreted as possibly relevant to all knee OA patients, regardless of their specific compartmental diagnosis.

A pooling of the available data on patellar taping from studies of its use in the treatment of nonspecific anterior knee pain and confirmed knee OA indicated that medially directed patellar tape was effective in decreasing chronic knee symptoms by 16.1 mm on a 100-mm pain scale (95% confidence interval [CI] 10.0–22.2 mm, $P<.01$) and 10.9 mm (95% CI 3.4–18.4 mm, $P<.01$) in comparison with no tape and sham taping, respectively. When limiting the analyses to only those studies involving subjects with diagnosed knee OA, the efficacy of patellar taping increased, resulting in pain decreases of 20.1 mm (95% CI 14.3–26.0, $P<.01$) in comparison with no tape, and 13.3 mm (95% CI 8.4–18.1 mm, $P<.01$) in comparison with sham taping. Although additional studies are needed to clarify the specific radiographic and physical findings that most strongly indicate its use, an examination of the current evidence suggests that patellar taping is effective in reducing chronic knee pain among patients with knee OA. The cost of the intervention is minimal, and the most serious side effects reported are local irritation of the skin. Although some older patients can be successfully taught to apply patellar tape themselves, frequent long-term use is unrealistic. If patients show a positive short-term response to taping, a comparable patellar brace should be sought for longer-term use.

Given the encouraging results about patellar taping, it is surprising that no published trials have yet examined the effects of patellar bracing (**Fig. 10**) among older persons with knee OA. It is to be hoped that the results of the recently completed crossover trial (Bracing in patellofemoral osteoarthritis: a clinical trial, DJ Hunter, PI, unpublished data, 2009) will help to fill this obvious void. Meanwhile, it may be necessary to infer the likely effects of patellar bracing on knee OA from studies of younger patients with nonspecific anterior knee pain. Among such studies, 3 trials (n = 119) compared patellar bracing with no bracing, and 2 trials (n = 94) compared patellar bracing with sham bracing. Pooling of data from this limited set indicated that patellar bracing was successful in decreasing pain by 14.6 mm (95% CI 3.8–25.5 mm, $P<.01$) in comparison with no bracing. However, patellar bracing did not differ in its measured effects from sham bracing ($P = .76$). Although it is not clear whether the observed effects of patellar bracing on nonspecific anterior knee pain also pertain to older patients with knee OA, the unpublished results of our own crossover trial suggest a comparable absence of effect when comparing patellar bracing with sham bracing among older adults with radiographically confirmed PF OA. If these preliminary findings are correct, the implication is that the substantial clinical benefits of patellar taping may not be so easily replicated using a PF brace. Alternative brace designs are being developed, and future trials are urgently needed to assess their effects among older patients with PF OA.

Patellar Brace
Anterior view

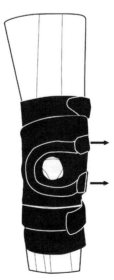

Fig. 10. Medially directed patellar bracing.

In light of the evidence supporting the efficacy of patellar tape in reducing pain among patients with knee OA, the clinician should feel confident introducing patellar tape as a safe and inexpensive, albeit impermanent, first line of therapy. Because there is currently no convincing evidence suggesting that patellar tape succeeds in markedly realigning the patella during weight-bearing knee function, or that the beneficial effects of patellar tape are limited to those patients whose knee OA remains confined to the lateral half of the PF compartment, patellar taping can be recommended as a treatment modality with potential application to lateral or medial PF OA, or to mixed TF and PF OA diagnoses.

Given the absence of any published clinical trials of patellar bracing among patients with knee OA, no firm guidelines for prescription can yet be derived. One method that has been helpful in the clinic is to select an activity, such as stair climbing or standing from a low chair, that is typically provocative of a patient's knee pain. The patient is asked to pay close attention to the intensity of their knee symptoms while repeating the aggravating activity with and without a generically sized patellar brace. If the brace is successful in improving knee symptoms, a prescription may be made on that basis.

VISCOELASTIC INSOLES AND THE HEEL STRIKE TRANSIENT

Each footfall during walking requires an abrupt deceleration of the limb at the moment that ground contact is made. Within milliseconds following initial contact, the GRF rises to a sharp peak and an impact shock wave is rapidly transmitted up the limb. Left unattenuated, the GRF, which, at the moment of initial ground contact is referred to as the heel strike transient, will pass jarringly up though the contacting heel and the tibia before eventually imparting a transient impulse to the tissues of the medial and lateral TF joint. The magnitude and frequency of this transient impulse depends on several external factors including gait velocity, stride length, and the compliance of the contacting ground surface. There are also several important internal mechanisms that serve to dampen and disperse the heel strike transient. The fat pad of the heel is one such mechanism. It has been proposed that the protective action of the cushioning fat pad may be supplemented with the addition of a viscoelastic insole. It is believed that these shock-absorbing insoles may be of particular benefit to older patients whose calcaneal fat pads may have thinned or whose lower extremity bones may have become more brittle and less compliant with age.

In the early 1970s, Simon and colleagues[43] and Radin and colleagues [44] proposed that repeated exposure to unabated heel strike transient forces might increase the risk of TF OA. This hypothesis was supported by findings from a series of animal studies that found that repetitive impulse loading, even at levels considerably less than the threshold for gross tissue failure, could eventually trigger pathologic changes in the articular cartilage[45,46] and subchondral bone.[47] Radin and colleagues[48] followed these animal studies with a small cross-sectional study of 18 human subjects with a history of recurrent knee pain (cases) and 14 age-matched subjects with no history of knee pain (controls). Biomechanical analysis of the subjects' walking pattern indicated significant group differences in the peak magnitude of the heel strike transient force and the peak magnitude of measured tibial deceleration during the same brief period. There were no group differences in self-selected walking velocity, stride length, or other parameters that might serve to confound the observed association. The presence of knee OA was not confirmed in any of Radin and colleagues' study subjects, and when a similar case-control study was performed among 9 subjects with radiographically confirmed TF OA, none of the previously observed differences were replicated.[49]

Thus, a causal link between the heel strike transient and TF OA remains to be convincingly demonstrated. To date, there have been no high-quality trials evaluating the effects of viscoelastic insoles on pain and function outcomes among patients with knee OA. Nevertheless, the possibility that viscoelastic insoles might help to relieve symptoms and reduce damaging impulse stresses at the knee should not be ruled out. Viscoelastic insoles made of silicone have been shown to markedly decrease the peak heel strike transient among healthy subjects.[50] In one randomized clinical trial involving 100 nursing students, these insoles also reduced weight-bearing–induced low-back pain.

Given their low cost and negligible risk profile, viscoelastic insoles can be safely recommended as part of a more comprehensive prescription for uni- or bicompartmental TF OA that may include athletic shoes with thick foam midsoles. In addition, encouragement should be given to patients whose symptoms are typically provoked with walking to concentrate on slowing the gait speed and making more gentle contact with the ground as they walk. This combination of interventions is often successful in improving tolerance for walking on noncompliant surfaces, such as asphalt or concrete.

LATERALLY WEDGED SHOE INSOLES AND GENU VARUM MALALIGNMENT

The apparent success of valgus-inducing unloader braces for the treatment of medial TF OA has invigorated efforts to develop less obtrusive interventions with similar realigning capabilities. However, interventions intending to unload the medial TF compartment using a laterally wedged shoe insole have so far not shown comparable success in the few well-controlled clinical trials that have examined their effectiveness.[51]

Laboratory studies indicate that laterally wedged shoe insoles probably do help to realign the malaligned genu varum limb, and thereby reduce the M_{add} that is responsible for concentrating compressive load on the medial TF joint (**Fig. 11**).[52] However, the magnitude of these changes tends to be small. Kerrigan and colleagues[53] found that, in comparison with no insole, 5 degrees of lateral wedging succeeded in reducing the peak M_{add} by only about 6%. Ten degrees of lateral wedging reduced the peak M_{add} by 8%. These findings are entirely consistent with those of Crenshaw and colleagues[54] who found that the M_{add} was reduced by 7% when walking with a 5 degree laterally wedged insole. Although desirable, such small reductions amount to only slightly more than half the reductions achieved in the M_{add} using a valgus-inducing unloader knee brace.

These small mechanical effects probably occur by way of slight alterations in the frontal plane alignment of the TF joint.[55] However, any resulting reductions in activity-related knee symptoms require a minimum of 5 to 10 hours of daily insole use,[56] and result in symptom improvements that are not much greater than the reductions achieved by placebo alone.[51,57] In 1 of only 2 randomized trials meeting the criteria for inclusion in a Cochrane-sponsored review,[25] Maillefert and colleagues[57] reported slightly reduced NSAID use (4 fewer days in 3 months) and slightly greater compliance among a group of subjects with medial TF OA who were assigned a 5 degree laterally wedged insole versus a comparison group that used a neutral insole. However, after 6 months there were no differences in pain or function scores between the 2 groups. Similarly, Baker and colleagues,[58] in a well-conducted crossover study of 90 subjects with medial TF OA, reported a mean difference in pain reduction in the 6-week treatment period (5 degree laterally wedged insole) versus the 6-week control period (neutral insole) equal to just 13.8 points on a 500-point pain scale (95% CI −3.9,

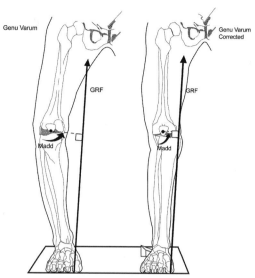

Fig. 11. (*Left*) Genu varum malalignment results in a large adduction moment (M_{add}) which concentrates compressive load on the medial TF compartment (*left*). The same limb with a laterally wedged insole (*right*) has improved TF alignment and a commensurate reduction in the adduction moment (M_{add}).

31.4). Comparably small and statistically nonsignificant effects were reported for all the secondary outcomes, including measured disability and several different physical performance tests.

Attempts to improve on the efficacy of laterally wedged insoles by increasing their inclination have met with only modest reductions in measured stress on the knee. The more pronounced effect of increasing the angle of inclination of the wedge is an increase in the number of new musculoskeletal complaints.[53] Any effort to significantly reduce painful compressive loading on tissues of the medial TF compartment by way of valgus realignment of the rearfoot also brings with it the unwanted risk of provoking problems related to excessive rearfoot pronation.[59] To the extent that excessive rearfoot pronation can adversely affect habitual loads on the knee, lateral heel wedges may, in the long run, lead to more harm than good among patients with preexisting foot hyperpronation. Thus, before any serious consideration is given to the use of laterally wedged insoles in the treatment of medial TF OA, the patient should be cleared for any significant history of preexisting foot or ankle problems, and a quick visual assessment should made of the patient's habitual standing and walking postures to rule out the presence of excessively flat or hyperpronating feet.

MEDIAL FOOT ORTHOSES AND FLAT FEET

Many conservative realignment therapies, including laterally wedged shoe insoles and unloader knee braces, are principally intended for treating only unicompartmental TF OA. Intuitively, if a realigning intervention succeeds in increasing joint space and reducing compressive load in the medial TF compartment, a coincident reduction of joint space and an increase in compressive load can be expected in the lateral TF compartment. As a result, many realigning knee interventions are contraindicated for patients whose knee OA is broadly symptomatic across medial and lateral TF compartments.

The principal intent of laterally wedged shoe insoles is to reduce genu varum malalignment and thereby minimize medial TF loading among patients with unicompartmental medial TF OA. Therefore, it might reasonably be expected that medially wedged shoe insoles should be similarly intended only for patients with genu valgum malalignment and unicompartmental lateral TF OA. Consistent with these expectations, the results of a randomized controlled trial by Rodrigues and colleagues[60] confirmed that insoles with medial heel wedging can produce substantial clinical improvements among patients with isolated lateral TF disease. Among 30 patients with unicompartmental lateral TF OA and genu valgum malalignment, Rodrigues and colleagues[60] found significant group differences on all measured clinical outcomes, including pain at rest, pain during movement, pain at night, and total Western Ontario and McMaster Universities Osteoarthritis Index (WOMAC) and Lequesne index scores after 8 weeks of an 8-mm medial heel wedge (n = 16) or a flat insole made of the same material (n = 14). Coincident reductions in standing genu valgum malalignment within the treatment group suggested that the probable mechanism of action involved the expected increases in lateral TF joint space and reductions in lateral TF compressive loading.

However, not all medial foot orthoses consist of only medial heel wedges. Among a diverse class of medial foot orthoses intended for persons with excessively flat feet, there exists an enormous variety of design features and construction materials that can be modified and customized to variously affect the frontal, sagittal, and transverse plane kinematics of the limb while simultaneously augmenting or restricting the foot's shock-absorbing capabilities. Few of the clinical findings that might indicate whether a particular orthotic design is preferable have been adequately clarified, least of all for knee disorders.

Numerous studies have investigated the effects of pes planus (flat feet) and pes cavus (high arched feet) on the occurrence of overuse injuries in the lower extremity, including chronic knee pain, iliotibial band syndrome, and patellar tendonitis.[61–64] However, the results of these studies are often inconsistent. For example, Dahle and colleagues[61] found that adults with pes planus or pes cavus experienced higher incidences of knee pain than adults with neutral foot alignment. In contrast, Cowan and colleagues[62] found that only adults with pes cavus had an increased risk of knee injury, whereas adults with pes planus had a reduced risk of knee injury. Kaufman and colleagues[63] found no association between foot alignment and knee pain, whereas Williams and colleagues[64] found that the pattern of overuse injury among active younger adults with low arches tended to differ substantially from the pattern typically exhibited by those with high arches. Among the most common injuries experienced by active younger adults with pes planus were patellar tendonitis and chronic knee pain.

The author is aware of only 2 studies that have specifically examined the relationship between flat-footedness and knee pain among older adults. Reilly and colleagues[65] found significant differences in foot alignment among 3 groups of patients: those with symptomatic medial TF OA, those with hip OA, and a control group consisting of age-matched older adults. In comparison with the other 2 groups, patients with medial TF OA had diminished arch height and more-severe rearfoot pronation in standing. Similarly, in a study of 1903 unselected older adults in the Framingham Study,[66] it was found that limbs with the most planus feet in standing had 1.3

(95%CI 1.1, 1.6) times the odds of frequent knee pain (P = .009), and 1.4 (95%CI 1.1, 1.8) times the odds of medial TF cartilage damage (P = .002) as limbs with the least planus feet. That these associations persisted even after adjusting for the presence of genu varum or valgum malalignment suggests that flat-footedness may be linked to heightened mechanical stress on the knee by mechanisms other than those involving only frontal plane knee malalignment. Previous theorists have posited that the transverse plane limb motions that accompany excessive foot pronation are likely to increase shear stress on the TF joint and increase the tendency for lateral maltracking of the patella.

If a patient with symptomatic knee OA presents with markedly flat feet, then improvements to foot alignment may result from interventions, such as medial foot orthoses, that are designed to limit pronation. By improving foot alignment, it is hoped that many related abnormalities of knee posture and motion will also improve. Although the findings of Rodrigues and colleagues[60] have begun to provide clearer evidence in support of using simple medial heel wedges to treat unicompartmental lateral TF OA, there is still a paucity of available research to clarify the appropriate role of antipronatory medial foot orthoses in treating symptomatic knee OA. Clinical experience suggests that medial foot orthoses may have much broader application to the treatment of a symptomatic OA in several different knee compartments. Although a meta-analysis[67] has confirmed the value of medial foot orthoses in preventing a wide variety of lower extremity overuse injuries among younger adults (pooled rate ratio [RR] = 1.5 [95% CI 1.1, 2.1]), no randomized clinical trials have yet studied the effectiveness of medial foot orthoses in reducing knee pain among older adults with flat feet and knee OA.

An approach that holds great promise was described in a pilot study[68] in which 15 older adults (24 knees) with medial TF OA and pes planus were treated using a

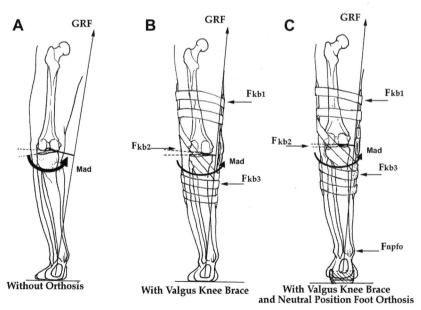

Fig. 12. Posterior view of lower limb: (*A*) genu varum malalignment with excessively pronated foot; (*B*) the same limb with a valgus unloader knee brace; (*C*) the same limb with a valgus unloader knee brace and a medial foot orthosis.

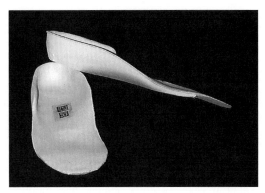

Fig. 13. Full-length custom-molded foot orthosis with shock-absorbent material, deep heel cup, and medial longitudinal arch support. The custom-molded foot orthosis is made from a foot impression (eg, plaster slipper cast) and, in this case, a trilaminate of materials supplying support, realignment, and shock absorption to selected regions of the foot.

valgus-inducing unloader knee brace and a customized antipronatory medial foot orthosis (**Fig. 12**). The patients were randomly assigned to 1 of 2 treatment groups. The first group was treated with a valgus-inducing unloader knee brace only, whereas the second group was treated using the combination of a valgus-inducing unloader knee brace and a customized medial foot orthosis. Although both groups showed decreased knee pain and improved function after 3 months, the group receiving the combined prescription had significantly greater improvements than the group treated with the knee brace alone. Based on these preliminary findings and increasing clinical experience, interventions that combine knee and foot orthoses may be used to good effect, especially among patients exhibiting medial TF OA and excessive foot pronation.

As with knee braces, over-the-counter foot orthoses are typically only available in discrete sizes (eg, small, medium, and large) and are often made of lighter duty, albeit less expensive, materials than their custom-molded counterparts. However, some orthotic designs may be significantly more effective than others.[69,70] A full-length custom-molded foot orthosis is shown in **Fig. 13**. The orthosis is made from shock-absorbent material, has a deep heel cup, and has a medial longitudinal arch support. A custom-molded foot orthosis is typically constructed by taking a foot impression (eg, plaster slipper cast) and then molding an orthosis to fit that impression. Additional

Table 1 Brace and orthotic considerations for managing OA in various knee compartments	
PF OA	Consider patellar taping for short-term management Evaluate response to patellar bracing for long-term management Consider a custom-molded foot orthosis to control excessive foot pronation
Medial TF OA	Consider a valgus-inducing unloader knee brace with or without a custom-molded foot orthosis to control excessive foot pronation and temper shock
Lateral TF OA	Consider a varus-inducing unloader knee brace with or without a custom-molded foot orthosis to control excessive foot pronation Consider a medial heel wedge

material is added to the orthosis to provide support, realignment, and shock absorption for selected areas of the foot.

SUMMARY

Based on the current literature and my clinical experience, I recommend the approach summarized in **Table 1** for treating knee OA using noninvasive knee and foot orthoses. As more research is completed in this understudied area, modifications and amendments to these suggestions will be necessary to integrate new evidence into clinical practice. The revaluing of conservative care strategies that make frequent use of noninvasive devices is a justifiable imperative for the future medical management of knee OA.

REFERENCES

1. Lawrence R, Helmick C, Arnett F, et al. Estimates of the prevalence of arthritis and selected musculoskeletal disorders in the United States. Arthritis Rheum 1998; 41(5):778–99.
2. Centers for Disease Control and Prevention. Arthritis prevalence and activity limitations – United States, 1990. In: MMWR Morb Mortal Wkly Rep 1994;43:433–8.
3. Third National Health and Nutrition Examination Survey (NHANES III). In: Centers for Disease Control and Prevention; 1993–1994. Available at: http://www.cdc.gov/nchs/NHANES.htm. Accessed March 31, 2010.
4. Burden of musculoskeletal diseases in the United States: prevalence, societal and economic cost. Rosemont (IL): American Academy of Orthopaedic Surgeons; 2008.
5. Arthritis in Canada: an ongoing challenge. Ottawa: Health Canada; 2003 (Cat. #H39-4/ 14-2003E).
6. Guccione A, Felson D, Anderson J, et al. The effects of specific medical conditions on the functional limitations of elders in the Framingham Study. Am J Public Health 1994;84(3):351–8.
7. Ofman JJ, MacLean CH, Straus WL, et al. A metaanalysis of severe upper gastrointestinal complications of nonsteroidal antiinflammatory drugs. J Rheumatol 2002;29(4):804–12.
8. Ortiz E. Market withdrawal of Vioxx: is it time to rethink the use of COX-2 inhibitors? J Manag Care Pharm 2004;10(6):551–4.
9. Smalley WE, Griffin MR, Fought RL, et al. Excess costs from gastrointestinal disease associated with nonsteroidal anti-inflammatory drugs. J Gen Intern Med 1996;11(8):461–9.
10. Hochberg MC, Perlmutter DL, Hudson JI, et al. Preferences in the management of osteoarthritis of the hip and knee: results of a survey of community-based rheumatologists in the United States. Arthritis Care Res 1996;9(3):170–6.
11. Willson J, Torry MR, Decker MJ, et al. Effects of walking poles on lower extremity gait mechanics. Med Sci Sports Exerc 2001;33(1):142–7.
12. Kemp G, Crossley KM, Wrigley TV, et al. Reducing joint loading in medial knee osteoarthritis: shoes and canes. Arthritis Rheum 2008;59(5):609–14.
13. Andriacchi TP. Dynamics of knee malalignment. Orthop Clin North Am 1994; 25(3):395–403.
14. Recommendations for the medical management of osteoarthritis of the hip and knee: 2000 update. American College of Rheumatology Subcommittee on Osteoarthritis Guidelines. Arthritis Rheum 2000;43(9):1905–15.

15. Pendleton A, Arden N, Dougados M, et al. EULAR recommendations for the management of knee osteoarthritis: report of a task force of the Standing Committee for International Clinical Studies Including Therapeutic Trials (ESCISIT). Ann Rheum Dis 2000;59(12):936–44.

16. Neumann DA. Biomechanical analysis of selected principles of hip joint protection. Arthritis Care Res 1989;2(4):146–55.

17. Tetsworth K, Paley D. Malalignment and degenerative arthropathy. Orthop Clin North Am 1994;25(3):367–77.

18. Sharma L, Song J, Felson DT, et al. The role of knee alignment in disease progression and functional decline in knee osteoarthritis. Jama 2001;286(2):188–95.

19. Kraus VB, Vail TP, Worrell T, et al. A comparative assessment of alignment angle of the knee by radiographic and physical examination methods. Arthritis Rheum 2005;52(6):1730–5.

20. Chang A, Hayes K, Dunlop D, et al. Thrust during ambulation and the progression of knee osteoarthritis. Arthritis Rheum 2004;50(12):3897–903.

21. Ramsey DK, Briem K, Axe MJ, et al. A mechanical theory for the effectiveness of bracing for medial compartment osteoarthritis of the knee. J Bone Joint Surg Am 2007;89(11):2398–407.

22. Komistek RD, Dennis DA, Northcut EJ, et al. An in vivo analysis of the effectiveness of the osteoarthritic knee brace during heel-strike of gait. J Arthroplasty 1999;14(6):738–42.

23. Lindenfeld TN, Hewett TE, Andriacchi TP. Joint loading with valgus bracing in patients with varus gonarthrosis. Clin Orthop Relat Res 1997;(344):290–7.

24. Pollo FE, Otis JC, Backus SI, et al. Reduction of medial compartment loads with valgus bracing of the osteoarthritic knee. Am J Sports Med 2002;30(3):414–21.

25. Brouwer RW, Jakma TS, Verhagen AP, et al. Braces and orthoses for treating osteoarthritis of the knee. Cochrane Database Syst Rev 2005;(1);CD004020.

26. Kirkley A, Webster-Bogaert S, Litchfield R, et al. The effect of bracing on varus gonarthrosis. J Bone Joint Surg Am 1999;81(4):539–48.

27. Brouwer RW, van Raaij TM, Verhaar JA, et al. Brace treatment for osteoarthritis of the knee: a prospective randomized multi-centre trial. Osteoarthritis Cartilage 2006;14(8):777–83.

28. Hinman RS, Crossley KM. Patellofemoral joint osteoarthritis: an important subgroup of knee osteoarthritis. Rheumatology (Oxford) 2007;46(7):1057–62.

29. Zhang Y, Xu L, Nevitt MC, et al. Comparison of the prevalence of knee osteoarthritis between the elderly Chinese population in Beijing and whites in the United States: the Beijing Osteoarthritis Study. Arthritis Rheum 2001;44(9):2065–71.

30. McAlindon TE, Snow S, Cooper C, et al. Radiographic patterns of osteoarthritis of the knee joint in the community: the importance of the patellofemoral joint. Ann Rheum Dis 1992;51(7):844–9.

31. Duncan RC, Hay EM, Saklatvala J, et al. Prevalence of radiographic osteoarthritis–it all depends on your point of view. Rheumatology (Oxford) 2006;45(6): 757–60.

32. Perry J. Gait analysis: normal and pathological function. Thorofare (NJ): Slack, Inc; 1992.

33. Walker CR, Myles C, Nutton R, et al. Movement of the knee in osteoarthritis. The use of electrogoniometry to assess function. J Bone Joint Surg Br 2001;83(2): 195–8.

34. Rowe PJ, Myles CM, Walker C, et al. Knee joint kinematics in gait and other functional activities measured using flexible electrogoniometry: how much knee motion is sufficient for normal daily life? Gait Posture 2000;12(2):143–55.

35. Costigan PA, Deluzio KJ, Wyss UP. Knee and hip kinetics during normal stair climbing. Gait Posture 2002;16(1):31–7.
36. Grelsamer RP, Weinstein CH. Applied biomechanics of the patella. Clin Orthop Relat Res 2001;(389):9–14.
37. Besier TF, Draper CE, Gold GE, et al. Patellofemoral joint contact area increases with knee flexion and weight-bearing. J Orthop Res 2005;23(2):345–50.
38. Lesher JD, Sutlive TG, Miller GA, et al. Development of a clinical prediction rule for classifying patients with patellofemoral pain syndrome who respond to patellar taping. J Orthop Sports Phys Ther 2006;36(11):854–66.
39. Gigante A, Pasquinelli FM, Paladini P, et al. The effects of patellar taping on patellofemoral incongruence. A computed tomography study. Am J Sports Med 2001;29(1):88–92.
40. Powers CM, Heino JG, Rao S, et al. The influence of patellofemoral pain on lower limb loading during gait. Clin Biomech (Bristol, Avon) 1999;14(10):722–8.
41. Powers CM, Ward SR, Chan LD, et al. The effect of bracing on patella alignment and patellofemoral joint contact area. Med Sci Sports Exerc 2004;36(7):1226–32.
42. Warden SJ, Hinman RS, Watson MA Jr, et al. Patellar taping and bracing for the treatment of chronic knee pain: a systematic review and meta-analysis. Arthritis Rheum 2008;59(1):73–83.
43. Simon S, Radin EL, Paul IL, et al. The response of joints to impact loading. II. In vivo behavior of subchondral bone. J Biomech 1972;5(3):267–72.
44. Radin E, Parker HG, Pugh JW, et al. Response of joints to impact loading. 3. Relationship between trabecular microfractures and cartilage degeneration. J Biomech 1973;6(1):51–7.
45. Radin EL, Ehrlich MG, Chernack R, et al. Effect of repetitive impulsive loading on the knee joints of rabbits. Clin Orthop Relat Res 1978;(131):288–93.
46. Radin EL, Orr RB, Kelman JL, et al. Effect of prolonged walking on concrete on the knees of sheep. J Biomech 1982;15(7):487–92.
47. Burr DB, Radin EL. Microfractures and microcracks in subchondral bone: are they relevant to osteoarthrosis? Rheum Dis Clin North Am 2003;29(4):675–85.
48. Radin EL, Yang KH, Riegger C, et al. Relationship between lower limb dynamics and knee joint pain. J Orthop Res 1991;9(3):398–405.
49. Henriksen M, Simonsen EB, Graven-Nielsen T, et al. Impulse-forces during walking are not increased in patients with knee osteoarthritis. Acta Orthop 2006;77(4):650–6.
50. Folman Y, Wosk J, Shabat S, et al. Attenuation of spinal transients at heel strike using viscoelastic heel insoles: an in vivo study. Prev Med 2004;39(2):351–4.
51. Pham T, Maillefert JF, Hudry C, et al. Laterally elevated wedged insoles in the treatment of medial knee osteoarthritis. A two-year prospective randomized controlled study. Osteoarthritis Cartilage 2004;12(1):46–55.
52. Ogata K, Yasunaga M, Nomiyama H. The effect of wedged insoles on the thrust of osteoarthritic knees. Int Orthop 1997;21(5):308–12.
53. Kerrigan DC, Lelas JL, Goggins J, et al. Effectiveness of a lateral-wedge insole on knee varus torque in patients with knee osteoarthritis. Arch Phys Med Rehabil 2002;83(7):889–93.
54. Crenshaw SJ, Pollo FE, Calton EF. Effects of lateral-wedged insoles on kinetics at the knee. Clin Orthop Relat Res 2000;(375):185–92.
55. Toda Y, Tsukimura N. A 2-year follow-up of a study to compare the efficacy of lateral wedged insoles with subtalar strapping and in-shoe lateral wedged

insoles in patients with varus deformity osteoarthritis of the knee. Osteoarthritis Cartilage 2006;14(3):231–7.

56. Toda Y, Tsukimura N, Segal N. An optimal duration of daily wear for an insole with subtalar strapping in patients with varus deformity osteoarthritis of the knee. Osteoarthritis Cartilage 2005;13(4):353–60.

57. Maillefert J, Hudry C, Baron G, et al. Laterally elevated wedged insoles in the treatment of medial knee osteoarthritis: a prospective randomized controlled study. Osteoarthritis Cartilage 2001;9(8):738–45.

58. Baker K, Goggins J, Xie H, et al. A randomized crossover trial of a wedged insole for treatment of knee osteoarthritis. Arthritis Rheum 2007;56(4):1198–203.

59. Friedlaender GE, Strong DM, Tomford WW, et al. Long-term follow-up of patients with osteochondral allografts. A correlation between immunologic responses and clinical outcome. Orthop Clin North Am 1999;30(4):583–8.

60. Rodrigues PT, Ferreira AF, Pereira RM, et al. Effectiveness of medial-wedge insole treatment for valgus knee osteoarthritis. Arthritis Rheum 2008;59(5):603–8.

61. Dahle LK, Mueller MJ, Delitto A, et al. Visual assessment of foot type and relationship of foot type to lower extremity injury. J Orthop Sports Phys Ther 1991;14(2):70–4.

62. Cowan DN, Jones BH, Robinson JR. Foot morphologic characteristics and risk of exercise-related injury. Arch Fam Med 1993;2(7):773–7.

63. Kaufman KR, Brodine SK, Shaffer RA, et al. The effect of foot structure and range of motion on musculoskeletal overuse injuries. Am J Sports Med 1999;27(5): 585–93.

64. Williams DS 3rd, McClay IS, Hamill J. Arch structure and injury patterns in runners. Clin Biomech (Bristol, Avon) 2001;16(4):341–7.

65. Reilly A, Barker L, Shamley D, et al. Influence of foot characteristics on the site of lower limb osteoarthritis. Foot Ankle Int 2006;27(3):206–11.

66. Gross KD. Planus foot morphology is associated with knee pain and cartilage damage in older adults. Presented at the Annual Scientific Meeting of the American College of Rheumatology, 2008. San Francisco (CA), October 24–29, 2008. p. 701.

67. Collins N, Bisset L, McPoil T, et al. Foot orthoses in lower limb overuse conditions: a systematic review and meta-analysis. Foot Ankle Int 2007;28(3):396–412.

68. Hillstrom HB, Brower DJ, Bhimji S, et al. Assessment of conservative realignment therapies for the treatment of various knee osteoarthritis: biomechanics and pathophysiology. Gait Posture 2000;11(2):170–1.

69. Hillstrom HJ, Whitney K, McGuire J, et al. Evaluation and management of the foot and ankle. In: Robbins L, Carol S, Hannan MT, et al, editors. Clinical care in the rheumatic diseases. 2nd edition. Atlanta (GA): Association of Rheumatology Health Professionals; 2001. p. 203–11.

70. Hillstrom HW, Whitney K, McGuire J, et al. Evaluation and management of the foot and ankle. In: Bartlett CB S, Maricic M, Iversen M, et al, editors. Clinical care in the rheumatic diseases. 3rd edition. Atlanta (GA): American College of Rheumatology; 2006. p. 267–70.

Pharmacologic Intervention for Osteoarthritis in Older Adults

William F. Harvey, MD, MSc[a,b,*], David J. Hunter, MBBS, PhD, FRACP[b,c]

KEYWORDS

• Osteoarthritis • Geriatric • Pharmacology management

Osteoarthritis (OA) is the most prevalent form of arthritis and one of the leading causes of chronic disability among older individuals.[1] The health resource use imposed by OA is increasing because of the increasing prevalence of obesity and the aging of the community.[2] The largest increases will occur among older adults, for whom OA also has the greatest functional impact.

OA has been previously described as "degenerative joint disease". Although OA is characterized by degradation of the cartilage, this moniker understates the significance of genetic, biologic, biochemical, nutritional, and mechanical factors that contribute to the process.[3,4] Successful management of the disease requires a comprehensive approach to address all of these factors. In light of the potential for adverse events caused by the use of pharmacologic agents, the authors endorse the use of nonpharmacologic treatments before or in concert with pharmacologic therapy.

The focus of pharmacologic treatment of OA includes targets from the cell and cytokine level to the larger joint components such as cartilage, bone, innervations, and vascular supply. The intended important goals of therapy in patients with OA are pain management, improvement in function and disability, and ultimately disease modification. This articles discusses the current pharmacologic regimens available

Dr Harvey's work is supported by The American College of Rheumatology Research and Education Foundation Clinical Investigator Fellowship Award. Dr Hunter is supported by an ARC Future Fellowship.

[a] Division of Rheumatology, Tufts Medical Center, 800 Washington Street, Box 406, Boston, MA 02111, USA

[b] Division of Research, New England Baptist Hospital, 125 Parker Hill Avenue, Boston, MA, USA

[c] Department of Rheumatology, Northern Clinical School, University of Sydney, 2065, Sydney, Australia

* Corresponding author. Division of Rheumatology, Tufts Medical Center, 800 Washington Street, Box 406, Boston, MA 02111.

E-mail address: wharvey@tuftsmedicalcenter.org

Clin Geriatr Med 26 (2010) 503–515
doi:10.1016/j.cger.2010.03.008
0749-0690/10/$ – see front matter © 2010 Elsevier Inc. All rights reserved.

to address these goals. The review includes description of analgesic, antiinflammatory agents, injectables, and nutritional supplements. Specific attention is paid to current trends and controversies related to pharmacologic management, including the use of oral, topical, and injectable agents. In addition, there are 5 recently updated treatment guidelines for knee and hip osteoarthritis (American College of Rheumatology, Osteoarthritis Research Society International, American Academy of Orthopedic Surgeons, National Institute of Health and Clinical Excellence, European League Against Rheumatism).[5–10] Notations are made throughout the discussion highlighting which agents are recommended in these guidelines.

ANALGESICS

Symptom management in OA can be achieved with analgesic medications. These include drugs with various routes of administration as already discussed. Although symptom management does not alter the disease course, it can certainly lead to improvements in functional status and disability. Because delaying disease progression in OA is so challenging, ultimately moving a patient from being an individual with a painful joint, to being asymptomatic, may be the only realistic goal until the science of disease modification in OA is more advanced. Mitigating symptomatic concerns may lead to delay or deferred need of surgical intervention and thus potential reductions in the overall cost to patients and the health care system.

Acetaminophen (paracetamol) is the most commonly used analgesic for mild to moderate pain in OA.[11] Having no known disease-modifying properties, it is a pure analgesic, in contrast to nonsteroidal antiinflammatory drugs (NSAIDs) which have analgesic and antiinflammatory properties. The mechanism of action of acetaminophen is not well understood, but likely involves some modification of the cyclooxygenase system without affecting the inflammatory cascade. The drug is notable for its rapid onset of action (<1 hour) and short duration of action (4–6 hours).[12] It is metabolized by the liver and potentially toxic metabolites are excreted in the urine and therefore must be used with caution in patients with liver or kidney disease. Care should also be taken in patients who regularly consume even moderate amounts of alcohol as the liver toxicity of each can be synergistic. In standard doses the drug is usually well tolerated, causing few gastrointestinal (GI) or hematologic side effects.[13]

The use of acetaminophen as the first-line drug in mild to moderate OA has been controversial within the rheumatology community. Numerous studies have demonstrated its efficacy in reducing the pain of osteoarthritis.[14,15] Its status as a pure analgesic, however, has made it arguably less favorable than the NSAID class of drugs. This controversy has become more apparent because of the balance between the increasing recognition of the inflammatory components (such as the presence of synovitis and bone marrow lesions) of OA and the association of NSAIDs with significant toxicities (cardiovascular and others).[16,17] There are clearly large subsets of people for whom the relative safety of acetaminophen makes it a clear choice as the first-line agent for osteoarthritis. Acetaminophen in doses greater than 2000 mg/d and 2600 mg/d has also been associated with higher rates of GI adverse events.[18,19] In June 2009, a US Food and Drug Administration (FDA) advisory panel voted to recommend lowering the recommended daily maximum to less than 4 g/d, but the panel did not recommend a new maximum dose.[20] The FDA has not yet acted on the panel's recommendation. Therefore the role of acetaminophen in the treatment of OA requires a balance of potential toxicities, patient preference, and an understanding by patient and physician alike of the potential benefits. Acetaminophen is recommended in all 5 treatment guidelines (**Table 1**).

Table 1
Summary of guidelines for pharmacologic therapy for knee and hip osteoarthritis from 5 organizations by strength of recommendation

Pharmaceutical	ACR[6]	EULAR[8,9]	OARSI[10]	AAOS[7]	NICE[5]
Acetaminophen	1	1	1	1	1
Tramadol	2				
Opiates	2	2	2		2
NSAIDs	1	2	1	1	2
Cox-2	2	2	1	2	2
Topical NSAID	2	1	1	2	1
Capsaicin	2	1	1		2
Topical salicylate	2	1			NR
Intraarticular steroids	1	2	2	Short-term only	2
Intraarticular hyaluronic acid	2	2	2	NR	NR
Glucosamine and chondroitin		2	2	NR	NR

Abbreviations: 1, first line; 2, second line; AAOS, American Academy of Orthopedic Surgeons, 2008; ACR, American College of Rheumatology, 2000; blank, no opinion in the recommendations; EULAR, European League Against Rheumatism, 2003 knee, 2005 hip; NICE, National Institute of Health and Clinical Excellence, 2008; NR, not recommended for use; OARSI, Osteoarthritis Research Society International, 2008.

Tramadol is a nonnarcotic opioid analgesic that is useful in the treatment of moderate to severe pain in OA. Its mechanism of action is different from and synergistic with that of acetaminophen. Combination of this drug with acetaminophen allows a lower dose of tramadol with the same analgesic benefit. Tramadol interacts with the serotonergic, GABAergic, and noradrenergic systems centrally to produce its effect. Tramadol is metabolized in the liver and excreted in the urine, requiring dose adjustment in patients with renal and hepatic impairment.[21] It must be used with some caution in elderly patients because of central nervous system (CNS) depression and in patients with a seizure disorder or in combination with other medications that alter seizure threshold. Tramadol has been associated with increased risk of serotonin syndrome when used in combination with monoamine oxidase inhibitor and selective serotonin reuptake inhibitor medications. The most common side effects are nausea, flushing, and drowsiness. Like acetaminophen, tramadol is a pure analgesic with no disease-modifying properties. Its efficacy has been demonstrated in patients with osteoarthritis, but the authors recommend its use only in patients with contraindications to other drugs or when analgesic benefit is not fully achieved with other agents.[22] Tramadol is mentioned in only the American College of Rheumatology (ACR) treatment guidelines (see **Table 1**).

Narcotic-containing medications of varying potencies are available. Their efficacy in treating acute and chronic pain conditions is well established.[23,24] However, because of restricted prescribing, potential for CNS depression, addiction potential, and lack of disease-modifying effects, their use is not in the first line of pharmacologic management. Care must also be taken with the use of compounds that also contain acetaminophen to avoid toxicity. The American Geriatric Society recently stated that, with these caveats, opioid therapy is a potentially useful tool in the treatment of chronic pain.[25] The authors do not recommend the routine use of these medications for pain control in OA, however in patients with inadequate response or contraindications to other therapies, treatment with long-acting narcotic medications may be an option. When prescribing these medications, the use of a comprehensive institutional guideline (commonly called narcotics contracts) is an inexpensive and effective way to minimize the potential for abuse and to assist with regulatory oversight.[26] Opiates are recommended as second-line therapy in 4 of the 5 treatment guidelines (see **Table 1**).

NSAIDS

NSAIDs are a large group of drugs with analgesic and antiinflammatory properties. As discussed earlier, although OA is believed to be a noninflammatory disease, magnetic resonance imaging studies have demonstrated the presence of inflammatory type lesions including synovitis and bone marrow lesions.[16,17] Because NSAIDs have antiinflammatory and analgesic properties, and patients prefer them because of greater efficacy,[27] many rheumatologists consider these drugs the most important first-line agents in treatment of osteoarthritis. There is some evidence that these agents affect measures of inflammation in patients with OA.[28]

NSAIDs inhibit the cyclooxygenase (COX) enzymes that convert arachadonic acid into prostaglandins, a major mediator of inflammation. The 2 well-known isoenzymes of the COX enzymes (COX-1 and COX-2) are inhibited by various NSAIDs to varying degrees. The COX-1 isoenzyme is of particular importance in mediating the gastric toxicities of the NSAID class, whereas the COX-2 isoenzyme has been implicated in mediating the cardiovascular toxicity of the enzyme. COX-2 is only expressed in cells activated by inflammatory cytokines and is believed to be most relevant to systemic antiinflammatory effects.

There are 6 major classes of NSAID medications with a significant amount of individual variation in pharmacologic properties.[29] Although numerous preparations have been shown to be efficacious in treating OA, there is a large apparent variation in individual patient response to each drug. There is no clear clinical data regarding the relative potency of the various medications, although drugs such as indomethacin and diclofenac are anecdotally believed to be more effective. In clinical trials, all NSAIDs performed similarly, with persons reporting approximately 30% reduction in pain and 15% improvement in function.[30] In addition, there is no evidence that NSAIDs alter the natural history of the disease. Studies have controversially suggested that the reduction in pain that results in improvements in walking speed (and therefore increased joint-loading forces) may increase the risk of structural deterioration.[31,32]

Toxicity remains the most troublesome aspect of prescribing NSAIDs for the treatment of OA. The most common toxicity of NSAIDS is gastrointestinal.[33,34] Through inhibition of prostaglandin synthesis by COX-1 enzyme, NSAIDs cause increase rates of gastritis and ulceration. This risk is highest among patients with a previous history of ulcer or GI bleeding, more than 60 years of age, more than twice the normal dose of NSAID, concurrent use of corticosteroids, and concurrent use of anticoagulants.[35] Evidence from clinical trials indicates that primary prevention of adverse GI events can be accomplished with misoprostil and proton pump inhibitors.[36,37] H2 blockers such as famotidine have not been shown to prevent gastric ulceration with persons on concomitant NSAIDs.[38] COX-2 selective NSAIDS showed a relative risk reduction of 0.49 in large trials as distinct from use of standard NSAIDs but their use must be weighed against the potential for cardiovascular toxicity.[39] Proton pump inhibitors have the strongest evidence for healing and prevention of further ulceration.[40]

Nephrotoxicity is also a significant problem with use of NSAIDs and is mediated by prostaglandin inhibition at the afferent arteriole of the glomerulus and by interstitial nephritis through unclear mechanisms.[41,42] Both of these toxicities are usually self-limited and are associated more often with individuals with preexisting renal disease.

Cardiovascular complications are increasingly being recognized as a complication of NSAID use, particularly with the COX-2 selective medications. Inhibition of vasodilatory prostaglandins results in hypertension and coadministration with aspirin reduces the antiplatelet effects of aspirin. Early studies had shown a possible cardiovascular benefit of NSAIDs other than aspirin, however a more recent long-term study of celecoxib and naproxen shows an increase in cardiovascular events.[43] The American Heart Association and the American College of Cardiology have each published guidelines recommending extreme caution when COX-2 selective NSAIDs are used in patients who have or are at risk for cardiovascular disease.[44] There are numerous ongoing studies to further examine this relationship. The authors currently use COX-2 selective agents only in patients with low cardiovascular risk and who have another indication, such as documented GI toxicity from nonselective NSAIDs, or concomitant warfarin use.

Despite toxicities, NSAIDs have been and will continue to be an important component of pharmacologic management of OA. Our current practice is to prescribe nonselective NSAIDs, often nonacetylated salicylates (such as salsalate or choline magnesium trisalicylate) as our first choice. If patients do not tolerate this drug, switching to another NSAID of a different class may be an effective alternative before moving away from NSAIDs as a whole. NSAIDs should be prescribed at their lowest effective dose. NSAIDs are part of all 5 treatment guidelines (see **Table 1**).

TOPICAL AGENTS

Topical agents are gaining in popularity because of the recognized toxicity of oral agents. Study of these medications has largely been restricted to small randomized trials of short duration. Thus the medications have only been proved suitable for short-term use for mild to moderate pain in OA.

Topical NSAIDs have been studied and are available. Topical diclofenac diethylamine gel has been shown to provide good short-term pain relief, with less GI and renal toxicity than oral diclofenac.[45,46] Topical NSAIDs are effective in relieving pain in OA compared with placebo for hand and knee OA.[45,47] Diclofenac sodium gel was recently approved for use in the United States after studies demonstrated efficacy with a dose of 4 g/d for knee OA and 2 g/d for hand OA.[48,49] In the United States, the main difficulty with the clinical use of this newer medication is cost. In most other countries, these are generically available over the counter. This drug represents a potential alternative for use in patients in whom there is concern about systemic toxicity of NSAIDs. Topical NSAIDs are recommended in all 5 treatment guidelines (see **Table 1**).

Topical salicylate-containing compounds work as rubefacients that presumably reduce pain through increasing local blood flow. Studies involving these agents also show only short-term benefit.[50] Examples include methyl salicylate, diethylamine salicylate, and hydroxyethylsalicylate and several are available over the counter in the United States. These medications, like topical NSAIDs, provide an alternative to systemically absorbed compounds. The main side effects are local skin irritation and strong odor. Topical salicylates are not recommended for use by one guideline, and are second line in another (see **Table 1**).

Capsaicin-containing products contain the oil extract form hot pepper plants. Application of capsaicin to the skin results in a burning sensation, which can be severe. It is proposed that the neurologic stimulus caused by this local irritation depletes substance P in the sensory nerve fibers. Substance P is a powerful pain stimulus and therefore its depletion results in generalized pain sensitization in the local area.

It has been shown to be effective for hand and knee OA.[51] Capsaicin in a concentration of 0.025% is better tolerated than 0.075%. This should be applied 3 to 4 times per day for at least 3 to 4 weeks for an adequate trial. A randomized controlled trial (RCT) showed capsaicin (0.075%) reduced pain and tenderness in patients with hand OA compared with placebo for 4 weeks.[52] A similar study in patients with knee OA produced similar results, with 80% of patients treated with capsaicin (0.025%) experiencing pain relief after 2 weeks.[53] Skin irritation is the major side effect, and accidental application to any mucous membrane, including eyes, nose, mouth, and genitals causes marked irritation; thus careful counseling of the patient is essential. Capsaicin is recommended in 4 of the 5 treatment guidelines (see **Table 1**).

Topical lidocaine has been used to treat the pain in OA, particularly in OA of the spine.[54] Lidocaine depolarizes the sensory nerve fibers rendering them unable to transmit pain signals. Commercial patches are expensive, but gels and creams can be used effectively in some patients if applied under occlusive dressings. This agent is not mentioned in any treatment guideline.

INTRAARTICULAR CORTICOSTEROIDS

There is a long history of injection of steroids into joints for the purpose of pain relief and antiinflammatory effect. Many studies show the efficacy of various preparations.[55] Although OA is not primarily an inflammatory disease, there are some inflammatory features and there does seem to be response in OA patients to antiinflammatory medications. Triamcinolone and methylprednisolone preparations are the most common, although there are others. In general, the authors believe the low-solubility compounds (such as triamcinolone hexacetonide) have a longer duration of action.[56] Despite this, clinical trials have not shown long-term benefits in patients with OA treated with intraarticular steroids and there is no evidence that injection of corticosteroids alters the natural history of the disease.[57] There is some evidence suggesting that they may have deleterious consequences on structure.[58,59] How this relates to frequency of use is unknown although current armchair wisdom suggests that no single joint should be injected any more than 4 times in the course of 1 year. Studies indicate that when otherwise not contraindicated, intraarticular corticosteroids are of short-term benefit (1 week only) for pain and function.[56] Thus, despite their widespread use to treat the pain associated with OA, patients should be counseled that the best evidence suggests minimal short-term benefit. Further, although clinical wisdom suggests that the presence of an effusion indicates likely therapeutic benefit, based on current data this wisdom is inaccurate.[60] Intraarticular corticosteroids are part of all 5 treatment guidelines (see **Table 1**).

HYALURONIC ACID

Hyaluronic acid has been suggested as a potentially disease-modifying drug for OA and has been investigated for OA of the hip, knee, ankle, and temeromandibular joint. In vitro and ex vivo studies have reported growth of cartilage in a dose-related fashion and suppression of interleukin 1β (IL1β)-induced metalloproteinases.[61,62] Indeed, 2 meta-analyses have been able to show statistically significant improvements in pain and function, although the degree of clinical response and duration of response were varied and furthermore most of the response was placebo related.[63,64] No study has been able to demonstrate a change in the rate of progression of disease. Furthermore, the meta-analysis by Lo and colleagues[64] suggests that the molecular weight of the compound may play an important role, with high-molecular-weight compounds showing better effect. A more recent meta-analysis that looked specifically at high-molecular-weight hylan versus low-molecular-weight hyaluronic acid showed a trend toward benefit of the larger compounds but also showed large heterogeneity between trials and more local adverse reactions to hylan.[65] This was recently confirmed in an RCT directly comparing these agents by the same group, supporting that there was little or no difference between high- and low-molecular-weight compounds in their efficacy but greater potential for adverse effects with hylan.[66] As with glucosamine and chondroitin, there is much variation between studies and the significant possibility of publication bias, making unbiased conclusions about intraarticular hyaluronic acid efficacy difficult. A recent meta-analysis indicated that compared with corticosteroids, hyaluronic acid injection for treatment of knee OA has a greater benefit that begins at 8 weeks and extends as far as 26 weeks.[67] Because of the high cost and modest benefit of these agents, as well as moderate rates of adverse events, the authors do not currently recommend clinical use of these compounds. Intraarticular hyaluronic acid is not recommended for use in 2 guidelines and is second line in 3 guidelines (see **Table 1**).

GLUCOSAMINE AND CHONDROITIN

Glucosamine and chondroitin as treatments for OA have received a great deal of attention and controversy. These compounds are important components of cartilage and theoretically, by increasing the level of these substrates, could aid in cartilage repair or slow cartilage destruction. At present, most of the controversy is about whether these agents have any proven efficacy for symptom or structure modification. A meta-analysis performed in 2005 indicated a modest benefit for glucosamine in reducing symptoms and slowing joint-space narrowing of the knee on radiographs.[68] Methodological concerns have been raised about many of the individual studies in this meta-analysis. When only trials with adequate blinding were analyzed, no benefit was found. Furthermore, the most positive studies were done using a proprietary glucosamine sulfate compound. Proponents of glucosamine use believe that this is more effective than glucosamine hydrochloride; opponents have raised concerns about industry and publication bias.[69] Resolution of this matter will likely require a nonindustry sponsored study of glucosamine sulfate as opposed to the recent expensive National Institutes of Health investment on the Glucosamine/Chondroitin Arthritis Intervention Trial (GAIT),[70] which found that glucosamine hydrochloride was no more effective than placebo but ultimately raised more questions than it answered because of concerns about the preparation used, the large placebo effect, and the multiple additional subset analyses performed. Until then, the authors conclude that glucosamine and chondroitin may be of potential benefit in treating the pain and function of OA, but widespread use of this expensive supplement is not endorsed until more transparent large-scale studies are completed. Glucosamine and chondroitin are not recommended for use in 2 treatment guidelines and second line in 2 guidelines (see **Table 1**).

NUTRITIONAL SUPPLEMENTATION

A great deal of research has been done on the nutritional aspects of OA. Numerous vitamin and mineral deficiencies have been linked with increase risk of OA and clinical trials are underway. Vitamin K was linked with the risk of OA, however a clinical trial of supplementation published in an abstract failed to show a benefit.[71,72] The trial included subjects with and without vitamin K deficiency and showed a trend toward significance in the group who were vitamin K deficient at baseline. Selenium has been shown to be a risk factor for OA, but no clinical trial has yet been done.[73] Vitamin D deficiency has been shown to be a risk factor for OA and 2 large clinical trials are ongoing to investigate its replacement on the development and progression of disease. Other antioxidant nutrients have been studied and discussed, including beta carotene, vitamin E, vitamin C (rose hip), and avocado soy unsaponifiables, with some suggestion that they may slow progression of disease but do not prevent its occurrence.[74] A more detailed review of nutritional risk factors for OA was published recently.[75]

EMERGING THERAPEUTIC TARGETS

There are a vast number of agents currently under development for the treatment of OA.[76] A comprehensive review of these targets was done by Dray and Read[77] and includes discussions of cytokines such as TNF-α and IL1β, receptors such as kinin, cannabinoid, and prostanoid receptors and numerous ion channels. In addition, an interesting new emerging therapy is a monoclonal antibody against the nerve growth factor inhibitor, tanezumab, which is currently in phase III clinical trials. Some attention is also being given to adjunctive therapies for chronic pain, such as antidepressants. The large number of potential therapeutic targets bring hope that treatment will move away from analgesia toward disease modification.

SUMMARY

Management of OA is focused on relief of pain and improvement of function. This is achieved through a comprehensive treatment plan including pharmacologic and non-pharmacologic therapies. In addition to the recommendations in this publication, there are many well-written guidelines available that describe the management of OA based on evidence from trials and expert consensus.[5-10] The ACR is currently updating their guidelines.

Pharmacologic management begins in most patients with analgesia using acetaminophen or NSAIDs, with careful attention to potential toxicities. In particular, the cardiovascular and GI toxicities of NSAIDs must be monitored carefully. Tramadol and narcotic medications can be useful adjunctive therapies. Topical NSAIDs, salicylates, and capsaicin can be useful as adjuncts or in patients for whom systemic medications are problematic. Intraarticular glucocorticoids should be reserved for the short-term management of acute pain flares with a note of caution given their short duration of effect and potential for long-term harm. Because of the continuing controversies and lack of clear beneficial evidence, glucosamine, chondroitin, and intraarticular hyaluronic acid should not be used routinely.

The future of OA prevention and treatment may involve nutritional supplements such as vitamin D or selenium, but conclusive trials have not been completed. Likewise, numerous potential targets for therapy are under intense investigation. However, the management of OA pain will continue to require a multifaceted approach and in the absence of agents that can modify the disease, should be the preeminent focus of clinical management.

REFERENCES

1. Centers for Disease Control and Prevention (CDC). Arthritis prevalence and activity limitations–United States, 1990. MMWR Morb Mortal Wkly Rep 1994; 43(24):433–8.
2. Badley E, DesMeules M. Arthritis in Canada: an ongoing challenge. Ottawa (Canada): Health Canada; 2003.

3. Felson DT. An update on the pathogenesis and epidemiology of osteoarthritis. Radiol Clin North Am 2004;42(1):1–9, v.
4. Martin JA, Buckwalter JA. Roles of articular cartilage aging and chondrocyte senescence in the pathogenesis of osteoarthritis. Iowa Orthop J 2001;21:1–7.
5. Osteoarthritis: national clinical guideline for care and management in adults. London: Royal College of Physicians; 2008.
6. Recommendations for the medical management of osteoarthritis of the hip and knee: 2000 update. American College of Rheumatology Subcommittee on Osteoarthritis Guidelines. Arthritis Rheum 2000;43(9):1905–15.
7. American Academy of Orthopaedic Surgeons clinical practice guideline on the treatment of osteoarthritis of the knee (non-arthroplasty). Rosemont (IL): American Academy of Orthopaedic Surgeons (AAOS); 2008. Available at: http://www.aaos.org/research/guidelines/OAKguideline.pdf. Accessed June 12, 2008.
8. Jordan KM, Arden NK, Doherty M, et al. EULAR Recommendations 2003: an evidence based approach to the management of knee osteoarthritis: report of a Task Force of the Standing Committee for International Clinical Studies Including Therapeutic Trials (ESCISIT). Ann Rheum Dis 2003;62(12):1145–55.
9. Zhang W, Doherty M, Arden N, et al. EULAR evidence based recommendations for the management of hip osteoarthritis: report of a task force of the EULAR Standing Committee for International Clinical Studies Including Therapeutics (ESCISIT). Ann Rheum Dis 2005;64(5):669–81.
10. Zhang W, Moskowitz RW, Nuki G, et al. OARSI recommendations for the management of hip and knee osteoarthritis, part II: OARSI evidence-based, expert consensus guidelines. Osteoarthritis Cartilage 2008;16(2):137–62.
11. Hochberg MC, Altman RD, Brandt KD, et al. Guidelines for the medical management of osteoarthritis. Part II. Osteoarthritis of the knee. American College of Rheumatology. Arthritis Rheum 1995;38(11):1541–6.
12. Clissold SP. Paracetamol and phenacetin. Drugs 1986;32(Suppl 4):46–59.
13. Graham GG, Scott KF, Day RO. Tolerability of paracetamol. Drug Saf 2005;28(3):227–40.
14. Altman RD, Zinsenheim JR, Temple AR, et al. Three-month efficacy and safety of acetaminophen extended-release for osteoarthritis pain of the hip or knee: a randomized, double-blind, placebo-controlled study. Osteoarthritis Cartilage 2007;15(4):454–61.
15. Shen H, Sprott H, Aeschlimann A, et al. Analgesic action of acetaminophen in symptomatic osteoarthritis of the knee. Rheumatology (Oxford) 2006;45(6):765–70.
16. Hill CL, Hunter DJ, Niu J, et al. Synovitis detected on magnetic resonance imaging and its relation to pain and cartilage loss in knee osteoarthritis. Ann Rheum Dis 2007;66(12):1599–603.
17. Hunter DJ, Zhang Y, Niu J, et al. Increase in bone marrow lesions associated with cartilage loss: a longitudinal magnetic resonance imaging study of knee osteoarthritis. Arthritis Rheum 2006;54(5):1529–35.
18. Garcia Rodriguez LA, Hernandez-Diaz S. Relative risk of upper gastrointestinal complications among users of acetaminophen and nonsteroidal anti-inflammatory drugs. Epidemiology 2001;12(5):570–6.
19. Rahme E, Pettitt D, LeLorier J. Determinants and sequelae associated with utilization of acetaminophen versus traditional nonsteroidal antiinflammatory drugs in an elderly population. Arthritis Rheum 2002;46(11):3046–54.
20. Nelson L. Summary minutes of the Joint Meeting of the Drug Safety and Risk Management Advisory Committee, Nonprescription Drugs Advisory Committee,

and the Anesthetic and Life Support Drugs Advisory Committee. Available at:http://www.fda.gov/downloads/AdvisoryCommittees/CommitteesMeetingMaterials/Drugs/DrugSafetyandRiskManagementAdvisoryCommittee/UCM179888.pdf. Accessed July 1, 2009.

21. Dayer P, Collart L, Desmeules J. The pharmacology of tramadol. Drugs 1994; 47(Suppl 1):3–7.

22. Cepeda MS, Camargo F, Zea C, et al. Tramadol for osteoarthritis: a systematic review and metaanalysis. J Rheumatol 2007;34(3):543–55.

23. Kalso E, Edwards JE, Moore RA, et al. Opioids in chronic non-cancer pain: systematic review of efficacy and safety. Pain 2004;112(3):372–80.

24. Markenson JA, Croft J, Zhang PG, et al. Treatment of persistent pain associated with osteoarthritis with controlled-release oxycodone tablets in a randomized controlled clinical trial. Clin J Pain 2005;21(6):524–35.

25. American Geriatrics Society Panel on Pharmacological Management of Persistent Pain in Older Persons. Pharmacological management of persistent pain in older persons. J Am Geriatr Soc 2009;57(8):1331–46.

26. Weaver M, Schnoll S. Abuse liability in opioid therapy for pain treatment in patients with an addiction history. Clin J Pain 2002;18(Suppl 4):S61–9.

27. Pincus T, Koch G, Lei H, et al. Patient Preference for Placebo, Acetaminophen (paracetamol) or Celecoxib Efficacy Studies (PACES): two randomised, double blind, placebo controlled, crossover clinical trials in patients with knee or hip osteoarthritis. Ann Rheum Dis 2004;63(8):931–9.

28. Brandt KD, Mazzuca SA, Buckwalter KA. Acetaminophen, like conventional NSAIDs, may reduce synovitis in osteoarthritic knees. Rheumatology (Oxford) 2006;45(11):1389–94.

29. Tannenbaum H, Davis P, Russell AS, et al. An evidence-based approach to prescribing NSAIDs in musculoskeletal disease: a Canadian consensus. Canadian NSAID Consensus Participants. CMAJ 1996;155(1):77–88.

30. Todd PA, Clissold SP. Naproxen. A reappraisal of its pharmacology, and therapeutic use in rheumatic diseases and pain states. Drugs 1990;40(1):91–137.

31. Blin O, Pailhous J, Lafforgue P, et al. Quantitative analysis of walking in patients with knee osteoarthritis: a method of assessing the effectiveness of non-steroidal anti-inflammatory treatment. Ann Rheum Dis 1990;49(12):990–3.

32. Huskisson EC, Berry H, Gishen P, et al. Effects of antiinflammatory drugs on the progression of osteoarthritis of the knee. LINK Study Group. Longitudinal Investigation of Nonsteroidal Antiinflammatory Drugs in Knee Osteoarthritis. J Rheumatol 1995;22(10):1941–6.

33. Flower RJ. Studies on the mechanism of action of anti-inflammatory drugs. A paper in honour of John Vane. Thromb Res 2003;110(5–6):259–63.

34. Flower RJ. The development of COX2 inhibitors. Nat Rev Drug Discov 2003;2(3): 179–91.

35. Lanza FL. A guideline for the treatment and prevention of NSAID-induced ulcers. Members of the Ad Hoc Committee on Practice Parameters of the American College of Gastroenterology. Am J Gastroenterol 1998;93(11):2037–46.

36. Scheiman JM, Yeomans ND, Talley NJ, et al. Prevention of ulcers by esomeprazole in at-risk patients using non-selective NSAIDs and COX-2 inhibitors. Am J Gastroenterol 2006;101(4):701–10.

37. Silverstein FE, Graham DY, Senior JR, et al. Misoprostol reduces serious gastrointestinal complications in patients with rheumatoid arthritis receiving nonsteroidal anti-inflammatory drugs. A randomized, double-blind, placebo-controlled trial. Ann Intern Med 1995;123(4):241–9.

38. Taha AS, Hudson N, Hawkey CJ, et al. Famotidine for the prevention of gastric and duodenal ulcers caused by nonsteroidal antiinflammatory drugs. N Engl J Med 1996;334(22):1435–9.
39. Silverstein FE, Faich G, Goldstein JL, et al. Gastrointestinal toxicity with celecoxib vs nonsteroidal anti-inflammatory drugs for osteoarthritis and rheumatoid arthritis: the CLASS study: a randomized controlled trial. Celecoxib Long-term Arthritis Safety Study. JAMA 2000;284(10):1247–55.
40. Lai KC, Chu KM, Hui WM, et al. Esomeprazole with aspirin versus clopidogrel for prevention of recurrent gastrointestinal ulcer complications. Clin Gastroenterol Hepatol 2006;4(7):860–5.
41. Abraham PA, Keane WF. Glomerular and interstitial disease induced by nonsteroidal anti-inflammatory drugs. Am J Nephrol 1984;4(1):1–6.
42. Huerta C, Castellsague J, Varas-Lorenzo C, et al. Nonsteroidal anti-inflammatory drugs and risk of ARF in the general population. Am J Kidney Dis 2005;45(3):531–9.
43. Hippisley-Cox J, Coupland C. Risk of myocardial infarction in patients taking cyclo-oxygenase-2 inhibitors or conventional non-steroidal anti-inflammatory drugs: population based nested case-control analysis. BMJ 2005;330:1366–9.
44. Bennett JS, Daugherty A, Herrington D, et al. The use of nonsteroidal anti-inflammatory drugs (NSAIDs): a science advisory from the American Heart Association. Circulation 2005;111(13):1713–6.
45. Lin J, Zhang W, Jones A, et al. Efficacy of topical non-steroidal anti-inflammatory drugs in the treatment of osteoarthritis: meta-analysis of randomised controlled trials. BMJ 2004;329(7461):324.
46. Niethard FU, Gold MS, Solomon GS, et al. Efficacy of topical diclofenac diethylamine gel in osteoarthritis of the knee. J Rheumatol 2005;32(12):2384–92.
47. Bookman AA, Williams KS, Shainhouse JZ. Effect of a topical diclofenac solution for relieving symptoms of primary osteoarthritis of the knee: a randomized controlled trial. CMAJ 2004;171(4):333–8.
48. Altman RD, Dreiser RL, Fisher CL, et al. Diclofenac sodium gel in patients with primary hand osteoarthritis: a randomized, double-blind, placebo-controlled trial. J Rheumatol 2009;36(9):1991–9.
49. Barthel HR, Haselwood D, Longley S 3rd, et al. Randomized controlled trial of diclofenac sodium gel in knee osteoarthritis. Semin Arthritis Rheum 2009;39(3):203–12.
50. Mason L, Moore RA, Edwards JE, et al. Systematic review of efficacy of topical rubefacients containing salicylates for the treatment of acute and chronic pain. BMJ 2004;328(7446):995.
51. Mason L, Moore RA, Derry S, et al. Systematic review of topical capsaicin for the treatment of chronic pain. BMJ 2004;328(7446):991.
52. McCarthy GM, McCarty DJ. Effect of topical capsaicin in the therapy of painful osteoarthritis of the hands. J Rheumatol 1992;19(4):604–7.
53. Deal CL, Schnitzer TJ, Lipstein E, et al. Treatment of arthritis with topical capsaicin: a double-blind trial. Clin Ther 1991;13(3):383–95.
54. Burch F, Codding C, Patel N, et al. Lidocaine patch 5% improves pain, stiffness, and physical function in osteoarthritis pain patients. A prospective, multicenter, open-label effectiveness trial. Osteoarthritis Cartilage 2004;12(3):253–5.
55. Arroll B, Goodyear-Smith F. Corticosteroid injections for osteoarthritis of the knee: meta-analysis. BMJ 2004;328(7444):869.

56. Bellamy N, Campbell J, Robinson V, et al. Intraarticular corticosteroid for treatment of osteoarthritis of the knee. Cochrane Database Syst Rev 2006;(2): CD005328.

57. Raynauld JP, Buckland-Wright C, Ward R, et al. Safety and efficacy of long-term intraarticular steroid injections in osteoarthritis of the knee: a randomized, double-blind, placebo-controlled trial. Arthritis Rheum 2003;48(2):370–7.

58. Behrens F, Shepard N, Mitchell N. Alterations of rabbit articular cartilage by intra-articular injections of glucocorticoids. J Bone Joint Surg Am 1975;57(1):70–6.

59. Papacrhistou G, Anagnostou S, Katsorhis T. The effect of intraarticular hydrocortisone injection on the articular cartilage of rabbits. Acta Orthop Scand Suppl 1997;275:132–4.

60. Jones A, Doherty M. Intra-articular corticosteroids are effective in osteoarthritis but there are no clinical predictors of response. Ann Rheum Dis 1996;55(11): 829–32.

61. Akmal M, Singh A, Anand A, et al. The effects of hyaluronic acid on articular chondrocytes. J Bone Joint Surg Br 2005;87(8):1143–9.

62. Waddell DD, Kolomytkin OV, Dunn S, et al. Hyaluronan suppresses IL-1beta-induced metalloproteinase activity from synovial tissue. Clin Orthop Relat Res 2007;465:241–8.

63. Arrich J, Piribauer F, Mad P, et al. Intra-articular hyaluronic acid for the treatment of osteoarthritis of the knee: systematic review and meta-analysis. CMAJ 2005; 172(8):1039–43.

64. Lo GH, LaValley M, McAlindon T, et al. Intra-articular hyaluronic acid in treatment of knee osteoarthritis: a meta-analysis. JAMA 2003;290(23):3115–21.

65. Reichenbach S, Sterchi R, Scherer M, et al. Meta-analysis: chondroitin for osteoarthritis of the knee or hip. Ann Intern Med 2007;146(8):580–90.

66. Juni P, Reichenbach S, Trelle S, et al. Efficacy and safety of intraarticular hylan or hyaluronic acids for osteoarthritis of the knee: a randomized controlled trial. Arthritis Rheum 2007;56(11):3610–9.

67. Bannuru RR, Natov NS, Obadan IE, et al. Therapeutic trajectory of hyaluronic acid versus corticosteroids in the treatment of knee osteoarthritis: a systematic review and meta-analysis. Arthritis Rheum 2009;61(12):1704–11.

68. Towheed TE, Maxwell L, Anastassiades TP, et al. Glucosamine therapy for treating osteoarthritis. Cochrane Database Syst Rev 2005;2:CD002946.

69. Vlad SC, LaValley MP, McAlindon TE, et al. Glucosamine for pain in osteoarthritis: why do trial results differ? Arthritis Rheum 2007;56(7):2267–77.

70. Clegg DO, Reda DJ, Harris CL, et al. Glucosamine, chondroitin sulfate, and the two in combination for painful knee osteoarthritis. N Engl J Med 2006;354(8): 795–808.

71. Neogi T, Booth SL, Zhang YQ, et al. Low vitamin K status is associated with osteoarthritis in the hand and knee. Arthritis Rheum 2006;54(4):1255–61.

72. Neogi T, Felson DT, Sarno R, et al. Vitamin K in hand osteoarthritis: results from a randomized clinical trial. Osteoarthritis Cartilage 2007;15(Suppl C):C228–9.

73. Jordan JM, Fang F, Schwartz TA, et al. Low selenium levels are associated with increased odds of radiographic hip osteoarthritis in African American and white women. Osteoarthritis Cartilage 2008;15(Suppl C):C33.

74. McAlindon TE, Jacques P, Zhang Y, et al. Do antioxidant micronutrients protect against the development and progression of knee osteoarthritis? Arthritis Rheum 1996;39(4):648–56.

75. McAlindon TE, Biggee BA. Nutritional factors and osteoarthritis: recent developments. Curr Opin Rheumatol 2005;17(5):647–52.

76. Hellio Le Graverand-Gastineau MP. OA clinical trials: current targets and trials for OA. Choosing molecular targets: what have we learned and where we are headed? Osteoarthritis Cartilage 2009;17(11):1393–401.
77. Dray A, Read SJ. Arthritis and pain. Future targets to control osteoarthritis pain. Arthritis Res Ther 2007;9(3):212.

Total Joint Replacement in the Elderly Patient

Carl T. Talmo, MD[a],*, Claire E. Robbins, PT[b], James V. Bono, MD[a]

KEYWORDS

- Osteoarthritis • Older adults • Total knee arthroplasty
- Total hip arthroplasty

Persons older than 65 years are categorized as the elderly or seniors. Those 85 years old and older are considered the oldest old. Seniors are the fastest growing population not only in the United States but worldwide. Approximately 605 million people worldwide were 60 years or older in the year 2000 and that is expected to increase and be close to 2 billion by 2050.[1] In 2050, children younger than 14 years will be outnumbered by seniors for the first time in history.[1,2]

The US Census Bureau confirms the number of Americans older than 65 years has increased by a factor of 12, from 3.1 million in 1900 to 38.9 million in 2008.[1,2] At present, 12.8%, or over 1 in 8 persons, is an older American.[3] By the year 2020, older Americans are anticipated to represent 17% of the total United States population, and by the year 2030 they will represent 20% of the population.[4,5] Patients older than 80 years who currently comprise more than 1% of the world's population are projected to comprise more than 4% of the world's population by the year 2050.[4,5] The fastest growing segment of the elderly population is the oldest old (85 years or older) group. In 2008, this group was 47 times larger (5.7 million) than it was in 1900.[3] This small segment of the population is projected to reach 19 million worldwide by 2050.[1]

This rapid increase in the elderly population is expected to have a significant impact on the utilization and economic burden of health care in the United States. This trend is particularly apparent in the cost associated with the treatment of musculoskeletal disease, as nearly 80% of the elderly population will present to their physician with a complaint related to the musculoskeletal system.[6]

Total joint arthroplasty has become an extremely effective and successful treatment for osteoarthritis (OA) of the hip and knee. The procedures are among the most

The authors did not receive any outside funding or grants in support of their research for or preparation of this work.

[a] Department of Orthopaedic Surgery, Tufts University School of Medicine, New England Baptist Hospital, 125 Parker Hill Avenue, Tufts University, Boston, MA 02120, USA

[b] New England Baptist Hospital, 125 Parker Hill Avenue, Tufts University, Boston, MA 02120, USA

* Corresponding author.

E-mail address: ctalmo@nebh.org

Clin Geriatr Med 26 (2010) 517–529
doi:10.1016/j.cger.2010.04.002
0749-0690/10/$ – see front matter © 2010 Elsevier Inc. All rights reserved.

successful treatments available to the elderly as quantified by several measures, including pain relief, improved walking, improved self care and function, and increased number of quality of life years gained.[7-17] There is also substantial evidence that elderly patients undergoing total joint arthroplasty receive these benefits along with an associated decrease in health care costs as compared with usual care.[18]

PREVALENCE OF HIP AND KNEE OSTEOARTHRITIS

While the exact etiology of OA remains poorly understood, the association between OA and aging is well documented.[4,5,19] Other risk factors include recurrent trauma, genetics, obesity, lifestyle, and occupational and other environmental exposures.[5,19,20] OA of the hip and knee typically causes significant and progressive pain along with deterioration in function, ambulation, and mobility, and is one of the leading causes of physical disability in the elderly population.[19] OA of the hip and knee is the most common musculoskeletal disorder to cause pain and disability in this age group, accounting for up to 60% of musculoskeletal complaints in the population older than 64 years in some reports.[6] An estimated 33% of persons between the ages of 63 and 93 years have radiographic signs of arthritis of the knees.[21] More specifically, 40% of patients 80 years or older show evidence of knee OA and almost 12% demonstrate radiologic changes of the hip.[19]

Total joint replacement (TJR) surgery provides pain relief and restores function in individuals with OA of the hip and knee. Advances in technology, surgical technique, and perioperative care over the past few decades have made total hip arthroplasty (THA) and total knee arthroplasty (TKA) more suitable for a wider age group of patients, including those older than 80 years.[9-11] Primary THA and TKA procedures increased steadily between 1990 and 2002, and the rate is projected to increase substantially over the next two decades.[22,23] Within the United States it is expected that the demand for THA will increase 174% by the year 2030, and TKA could reach as many as 3.48 million procedures.[21,23] The logistic and economic impact of these projections are far reaching, and will likely require a widespread understanding of the procedures and their perioperative care among all health care providers.

ECONOMIC BURDEN OF OSTEOARTHRITIS OF THE HIP AND KNEE

The anticipated economic impact of the aging population in the United States is substantial and multifactorial. Growth of the elderly population, the increasing volumes of primary and revision joint replacements, technological advances, increasing procedural and hospital costs, and the diminished reimbursement capacity of the Medicare system have created an economic burden.[21-23]

Approximately 93% of noninstitutionalized persons older than 65 years were covered by Medicare in 2007.[3] The Centers for Medicare and Medicaid services (CMS) pays for approximately 60% of the total joint arthroplasties in the United States.[21] About one-third of the associated procedural charges for revision total joint arthroplasty are reimbursed by Medicare.[21]

Annual hospital and surgical charges for total joint arthroplasties are estimated to show a significant increase by the year 2015, despite declining reimbursement to physicians and hospital over this same period. Technological advancements in prosthetic design to decrease wear and promote the longevity of the prosthesis are the most significant factors contributing to the increase in cost associated with the procedures over the last 20 years.[21,24,25] Combined hospital and surgical charges for primary THA and TKA are projected to be $65.1 billion by 2015.[22]

Iorio and colleagues[21] identify significant reimbursement discrepancies that may influence the retention and recruitment of orthopedic surgeons who perform primary and revision total joint surgeries. For example, the average physician payment for a total joint surgery declined 39% between the period 1991 to 2007. The CMS decreased physician payments by 9.9% in 2008 and the future reimbursement rates remain uncertain.[21] Innovations in technology, the rising cost of total joint implants, and other aspects of in-hospital and perioperative care have contributed to the economic burden, as Medicare and other health care payors have failed to reimburse hospitals at rates that are comparable to the rate of inflation.[21]

DIAGNOSIS AND REFERRAL OF PATIENTS WITH OSTEOARTHRITIS OF THE HIP AND KNEE

Pain in the area of the hip may have a myriad of causes, including degenerative arthritis of the hip or spine, bursitis, pain of a radicular origin, as well as referral from a hernia or intra-abdominal source. Pain coming from the hip typically originates in the groin and may radiate to the knee, thigh, or buttock area. The pain typically occurs with activity and ambulation, increases after periods of activity, and improves with rest. The pain may occur at night. Patients typically report some difficulty with self care, especially tying their shoes or putting on their socks. Physical examination findings in patients with hip OA include flexion and external rotation contractures and limitation in internal rotation, which is particularly evident in flexion. There may be a leg length inequality evident, and a limp with ambulation. The diagnosis is usually confirmed with plain radiographs, which show joint space narrowing, subchondral sclerosis, cyst formation, and osteophytes. Magnetic resonance imaging (MRI) scan is reserved for cases of unexplained pain or where avascular necrosis may be suspected. First-line treatment of hip OA includes acetaminophen or nonsteroidal anti-inflammatory drugs (NSAIDs), weight loss, and consideration for use of a cane.[20] Use of NSAIDs is associated with significant morbidity and toxicity in the elderly population, most notably a high rate of bleeding and peptic ulcer disease, and therefore must be monitored closely.[26] Patients at risk for NSAID-associated side effects are candidates for earlier referral and consideration for TJR.[18,20,26] Corticosteroid injections are reserved mainly for diagnostic purposes, and have little or no role in the treatment of chronic OA due to the associated risks of infection and progression of OA. Corticosteroid injections show limited benefits with essentially no improvement or alteration in the natural history of the disease. Use of cortisone in the hip joint carries a risk of infection, which can be devastating and may also contribute to the progression of OA as well as bony destruction to a greater extent than is seen in the knee or other joints (**Fig. 1**).[27] Patients with significant pain and functional disability due to hip OA are candidates for referral to an orthopedic surgeon for total hip replacement (THR). Other indications for THR in the elderly include rheumatoid arthritis (RA), osteonecrosis of the femoral head, acute femoral neck fracture, and nonunion or other complication following hip fracture surgery.

Pain caused by OA of the knee typically originates in the medial aspect of the knee, and may radiate anteriorly, posteriorly, or down the leg. The pain is exacerbated by walking or other physical activity as well as stair climbing, which is typically difficult as the disease progresses. There may be a history of injury or meniscal surgery. The patient may also report crepitation, buckling, or other mechanical symptoms. Angular deformities of the lower extremities are common, and the patient may report long-standing bowing deformity that significantly preceded the onset of symptoms. Additional physical examination findings include crepitus, flexion contracture, stiffness and limited motion, effusion, and joint line tenderness. Any evaluation of knee pain in the elderly warrants a clinical examination of the hip for referred pain, which typically is anterolateral but may also be medial. Plain radiographs of the knee are usually definitive for the diagnosis; however, hip radiographs may also be advisable if referred pain is suspected. In general, MRI scan has little value in the majority of elderly patients unless there is a suspicion of tumor or obscure infection, with negative radiographs and following failure of conservative measures, as the examination is overly sensitive and there is likely to be a high false-positive rate of meniscal tearing evident. Treatment of early knee OA includes acetaminophen or anti-inflammatory medications, weight loss in obese individuals, and assistive ambulatory aids. Physical therapy for quadriceps strengthening and water exercises may be beneficial.[19,20,28] Corticosteroid injection may be valuable for short-term relief of a painfully swollen arthritic knee, whereas viscosupplementation therapies remain controversial.[26] Patients with chronic symptoms and radiographic evidence of significant OA warrant referral for total knee replacement. Other indications for total knee replacement (TKR)

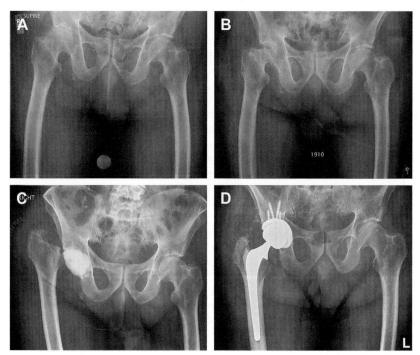

Fig. 1. A 76-year-old man presented with right groin pain and decreased walking tolerance. A radiograph (A) indicated joint space narrowing of the right hip and early degenerative changes. A radiologically-guided corticosteroid injection was performed, resulting in 1 week of improvement followed by severe increased pain. Repeat radiographs revealed rapid progressive joint destruction (B), and acute infection was suspected. Due to a high suspicion of infection despite a negative hip aspiration, the patient was treated with aggressive surgical debridement of the hip, placement of an antibiotic impregnated cement spacer, and intravenous antibiotics (C). Cultures and pathology specimens were subsequently negative for infection, and about 4 weeks later the patient underwent THR with a cemented femoral component utilizing antibiotic impregnated cement (D) for what is retrospectively presumed to be rapidly progressive OA following intra-articular cortisone injection.

include refractory RA or inflammatory arthritis, posttraumatic OA, or aseptic necrosis involving the knee.

Because of the progressive nature of OA in the hip and knee and the relative success of joint replacement surgery, early discussions with patients regarding future TJR are worthwhile. This education may help to allay patient fears and frustrations, and may avoid unnecessary overuse of health care resources and ineffective remedies.[8,18]

Contraindications to TJR are extremely rare and include active infection at the surgical site, extreme neuropathic disease resulting in a potentially flail extremity, extensive bone loss typically following prior joint replacement surgery, and extreme medical illness precluding anesthesia, typically where there is a significant risk of mortality even without surgery.[29]

EFFICACY OF TOTAL HIP ARTHROPLASTY IN THE ELDERLY

Modern THA, first performed in the early 1960s almost 50 years ago, continues to be one of the most successful interventions in medicine.[14,17,30,31] The procedure is essentially unrivaled in surgery in terms of its success rates and patient satisfaction.[17] Numerous studies have demonstrated improved pain, function, and quality of life following THR for several decades.[7–17,24,28] Using functional scoring systems and validated outcome measurements such as the short form-36 (SF-36) and the Western Ontario and McMaster University Osteoarthritis Index (WOMAC), several researchers have consistently shown significant improvement in health-related quality of life following TJRs, particularly with THR.[12–15] Improvement in SF-36 scores and other measures are significant when compared with preoperative scores, and the improvement has been shown to be superior to the improvement seen following TKR.[14–16] The degree of improvement in these scores for both hip and knee arthroplasty has also been shown to be significant and dramatic in effect when compared with traditional nonoperative or conservative measures.[11] Although comorbid illnesses can influence the results, this improvement has been noted across all age groups, and age has not been found to be an obstacle to successful surgery and outcomes.[8] Patients with a poorer preoperative health-related quality of life are also the most likely to experience a greater degree of improvement.[7,8,12]

Several studies have also demonstrated excellent results for THR in the elderly population, with low risks and complication rates.[10,32] Levy and colleagues[10] reviewed the results of THR in 100 patients older than 80, average age 85 years, undergoing THR for OA. At an average follow-up period of 5 years, 96% of patients maintained independent living and 98% were extremely satisfied with the procedure, while there was only one reoperation for a single infection. Another study by the same group demonstrated similar results at a minimum of 2 years' follow-up for a group of octogenarian patients who were deemed to be medically "frail" preoperatively.[29] Brander and colleagues[33] also demonstrated excellent pain relief and functional outcomes for THR in the octogenarian population, with the most dramatic improvement in function witnessed in the most disabled of this elderly group.

Patient satisfaction with TJR, particularly THR, in the elderly does not seem to be compromised in comparison with patients of a more youthful age group.[9,33–36] Pettine and colleagues[36] compared more than 100 hip replacements in patients older than 80 with a similar group of patients undergoing THR in their mid-sixties. These investigators found no statistically significant differences in pain or function at minimum 5 years postoperatively, although minor complications were twice as high in the older group and length of hospital stay averaged 2 days longer. In a large prospective study of Canadian patients, Jones and colleagues[34] noted excellent SF-36 and WOMAC scores in elderly and younger patients 6 months following TJR. After adjusting for confounding variables, there were no differences in joint pain or function in the elderly patients (older than 80) when compared with the younger group (age 55–79 years). The pain relief and functional improvements were significantly greater following THR when compared with TKR. The older patients were more likely to require an inpatient rehabilitation facility postoperatively. Longer-term follow-up studies have also demonstrated sustained improvements in pain and function as well as prosthesis durability in the elderly. Keisu and colleagues[37] reviewed the results of THR in 114 octogenarian patients at a mean follow-up interval of 5 years. Although 24% of these patients experienced a postoperative medical complication, there were no deaths related to the operation. At final follow-up, 25 patients had died; however, the average functional score for the remaining patients were in the good to excellent range and no patients required revision surgery at final follow-up.

EFFICACY OF TOTAL KNEE ARTHROPLASTY

TKA is one of the most highly successful and commonly performed orthopedic procedures in the United States. For the past 40 years, TKA has proven to be an efficacious treatment for persons with OA in relieving pain and restoring function.[8,12,15] Despite the success of the procedure and the fact that most patients undergoing joint arthroplasties are elderly (older than 65 years),[38] there remains hesitancy to perform this procedure on the oldest population and the frail elderly.[9,29,39,40] The changing demographics of the United States and worldwide populations show that the very elderly age group will outnumber those younger than 14 years within the next several decades. Mortality and complication rates from surgery are known to increase with this age group.[11] However, due to advances in technology, perioperative care, and rehabilitation, TKA is now an option for the very elderly and the frail elderly.[9]

There is extensive literature to support the efficacy of total knee replacement in the elderly.[4,9,11,29,34,39–41] Careful consideration should be paid to preoperative systemic disease, hearing or vision deficits, psychological status, living arrangements, and patients' expectations. With careful consideration and preoperative planning, treating the very elderly patient is typically safe and successful, and therefore advanced age should not be a limiting factor for knee replacement surgery.[29,34,39–41] Adam and Noble[42] retrospectively reviewed the results of TKR in a group of patients older than 75 years and noted excellent patient satisfaction, pain relief, stability, and range of motion comparable to a group of younger patients undergoing the procedure. Birdsall and colleagues[9] prospectively followed 119 patients older than 80 years after TKR and documented significant improvements in health outcome including improved pain, emotional reaction, sleep, and physical mobility as early as 3 to 12 months after the operation. Zicat and colleagues[35] compared 50 patients undergoing TKR after age 80 with 50 patients between the ages of 65 and 69 years in a prospective fashion. At a minimum of 2 years postoperatively, there was no difference between the groups in terms of pain, functional level, strength, stability, or range of motion, with significant improvement seen in both groups. The procedure was also equally cost-effective in both groups. In a retrospective study, Hosick and colleagues[43] found a higher rate of early postoperative medical complications in patients older than 80 years undergoing TKR, but still with significant pain relief and functional improvement following recovery.

In a prospective cohort study of patients undergoing TKR, evaluation preoperatively and 12 months postoperatively indicated SF-36 scores including function and measures of bodily pain equivalent to population norms for this age group. These results along with those from other similar studies indicate that age is not a risk factor for inferior outcome following TKR, and that elderly patients undergoing TKR function as well as patients of a similar age without OA.[12]

COMPLICATIONS AND SPECIAL CONSIDERATIONS FOLLOWING TOTAL JOINT REPLACEMENT IN THE ELDERLY

TJRs are relatively safe procedures with a low rate of complications in general. While there is some evidence that elderly patients may be at higher risk for medical and prosthesis-related complications following surgery, the evidence is conflicting. Smaller scale retrospective studies have indicated higher rates of mortality and complication rates in the elderly.[32,36,42–45] A larger scale study of Medicare claims data indicated that older age was a risk factor for an adverse outcome within 90 days following THR including death, dislocation, and infection.[31] Some reports indicate a higher rate of mortality, cardiopulmonary complications, hip dislocation, urinary tract infection (UTI), and other perioperative infectious complications following surgery in the elderly[31,32,46] Phillips and colleagues[45] reviewed perioperative complications in patients older than 80 years undergoing THR including death, postoperative myocardial infarction (MI), thromboembolism, urinary tract infection, and postoperative confusion, and found that complications and postoperative morbidity correlated significantly with the American Society of Anesthesiologists (ASA) score. Patients with an ASA rating of III or higher had a 15% risk of perioperative complication, significantly greater than those with an ASA class I or II.

More recent studies have demonstrated lower rates of postoperative complications across the board in TJR, most likely due to increased awareness and medical screening that has correlated with the increased volume of elective joint replacement occurring throughout the world.[31,34] In a review of more than 10,000 patients undergoing elective TJR, the overall rate of adverse events within 30 days of surgery was 2.2% including MI (0.4%), pulmonary embolism (PE) (0.7%), deep venous thrombosis (DVT) (1.5%), and death (0.5%), and the frequency of these events did increase with age, particularly for patients aged 70 years or older.[47] Other case-control and more comparative studies have found complication rates and mortality more comparable with those of other age groups undergoing TJR.[33–35] Complication rates in both groups certainly are low; however, based on these results, careful perioperative monitoring of elderly patients is warranted to aid in the prevention of complications. Certain potential complications in the elderly deserve special consideration so that appropriate prevention strategies may be employed without introducing additional morbidity, and are reviewed here in further detail.

Infection

Infection is a relatively rare yet potentially devastating complication following TJR. Infection rates vary from about 0.2% to 2.5% following elective TJR.[48–54] The risk of infection is slightly higher in TKR than in THR.[52] Risk factors for infection include age, diabetes mellitus, RA, a history of prior surgery on the joint, chronic infection elsewhere in the body, chronic kidney or liver disease, malnutrition, steroid use, smoking, and early wound complications or hematoma.[48–54] Other risk factors may include a higher ASA score, morbid obesity, bilateral surgery, allogenic blood transfusion, postoperative atrial fibrillation, MI, and prolonged hospitalization.[52]

There is increasing evidence that prolonged wound bleeding and drainage, hematoma formation at the surgical site, and reoperation for evacuation of hematoma places a patient at increased risk for deep infection.[53] For this reason, wound care and monitoring by the physician, nursing staff, and therapists is imperative following

TJR, and careful consideration must be given to postoperative anticoagulation along-side this.

Routine use of intravenous antibiotics covering gram-positive bacteria for preoper-atively and for the first 24 hours postoperatively has been shown to be preventative; however, continuing antibiotics beyond 24 hours has not been shown to be benefi-cial.[48] The most common pathogens identified in periprosthetic infections are skin flora including *Staphylococcus aureus* and *Staphylococcus epidermidis*, and therefore first-generation cephalosporins are the most commonly used prophylactic antibiotics.[50]

Periprosthetic joint infections may be superficial or deep; however, to avoid the devastating complication of chronic deep infection, all infections should be consid-ered deep until proven otherwise.[50] Routine administration of oral antibiotics for reddened wounds, a common finding after even uncomplicated joint replacement surgeries, is therefore discouraged in lieu of further careful assessment for signs of infection, possibly coupled with sterile joint aspiration and potentially more appro-priate surgical intervention where necessary.[50,53] The signs and symptoms of peri-prosthetic infection include increased pain, stiffness, prolonged or excessive wound drainage or dehiscence, and rarely, fever or constitutional symptoms as well. In the elderly or immunocompromised patient the presentation may be subtle until the infec-tion becomes severe and fulminant.[50,55]

The treatment of infections follows a fairly complex algorithm that typically involves surgical intervention for successful eradication.[50,55] Treatment of infections consid-ered superficial or acute includes surgical debridement with retention of the prosthesis and culture-specific intravenous antibiotics, whereas infections considered chronic and deep are treated with revision surgery in a single or 2-staged procedure followed by intravenous culture-specific antibiotics.[50,55] In the elderly patient with a poor life expectancy, chronic oral suppressive antibiotics alone or in combination with surgical debridement may be an appropriate treatment for sensitive low-virulence organisms, particularly when the risks associated with revision surgery are considerable.[50,55]

Thromboembolic Disease and Prevention

The incidence of DVT following TJR with prophylaxis is extremely low.[56] Following elective TJR with modern prophylaxis regimens the rate of symptomatic DVT varies around 1% to 2%, with a higher rate of DVT seen after TKR.[56] The rate of symptomatic PE with these regimens ranges from 0% to 0.5%, and is higher after THR.[56] Prophy-laxis against thromboembolism is therefore universally recommended. Agents commonly used in some combination include mechanical measures (thromboembolic deterrent compression stockings, lower leg or foot pneumatic compression boots), injectable low molecular weight heparins (LMWH), injectable synthetic pentasacchar-ides or factor Xa inhibitors, variable-dose warfarin, or fixed low-dose warfarin and aspirin.[56–58] Although a hypercoagulable state my exist up to 3 months following surgical intervention, most prophylaxis regimens are continued for only 10 days to 6 weeks postoperatively.[56] When choosing a regimen for prophylaxis, the surgeon must balance the risk of thromboembolism against the risk of bleeding and hematoma formation and the potential for infection at the surgical site.[57] Risk factors for throm-boembolic complications include a history of prior DVT or PE, advanced age, conges-tive heart failure, MI, stroke, obesity, and hypercoagulable states.[56,57] Easily overlooked when choosing a form of prophylaxis are preexisting risk factors for bleeding or hemorrhage, including history of bleeding disorder, gastrointestinal bleeding, hemorrhagic stroke, or other risks.[57] Elderly patients may be at higher risk for gastrointestinal complications or hemorrhagic stroke as well as having a higher potential for falls in the postoperative period, placing them at risk for soft tissue hematomas and intracranial or subdural bleeding.

The American Academy of Orthopedic Surgeons (AAOS), in coordination with other public health organizations, has therefore published practice guidelines based on a thorough review of the existing literature.[57] These recommendations support preoperative risk assessment for PE as well as bleeding and selection of a thromboprophylactic regimen that aims for a balance between safety and efficacy and balances anticoagulation and bleeding. Based on this balance, the AAOS has found that there is sufficient evidence to support the following chemotherapeutic regimens following TKR and THR: aspirin, LMWH, synthetic pentasaccharides, and variable-dose warfarin with a goal international normalized ratio of 2.0 or less.[57] For patients at higher risk of PE and a standard risk of major bleeding aspirin was not recommended, whereas for patients at a standard risk of PE and increased risk of major bleeding LMWH and synthetic pentasaccharides were not recommended, as these have been shown to result in an increased risk of bleeding, hematoma ,and wound drainage, which may influence the development of deep periprosthetic infection.[53,57] At their own institution, the authors have had success with a fixed low-dose regimen of warfarin (1 mg daily) for 6 weeks following elective THR in patients at standard risk for postoperative thromboembolism, obviating the need for blood draws with results comparable in terms of safety and efficacy with all other agents.[58]

Delirium

Postoperative delirium is a common and serious problem in hospitalized elderly patients following elective TJR.[59,60] Patients experiencing postoperative confusion and delirium can be disruptive and distressing to other patients and the health care team, but more importantly to themselves, frequently incurring self-inflicted injury or being susceptible to falls. Patients who have experienced delirium may have little or no recollection of the early postoperative period, and this loss of control is frequently disconcerting.[59] Delirium may occur in up to 44% of hospitalized elderly patients after major surgery[60] and in approximately 28% of elderly patients undergoing THR.[61]

The consequences of postoperative delirium including prolonged hospitalization, hip dislocation, immobility with associated skin compromise, infection and thromboembolic risk, falls and injuries, and the potential for impaired rehabilitation and recovery, are significant and may be costly to hospitals and the health care system.[59-62] Costs associated with the treatment of postoperative delirium have been estimated at 2.5 times that for other patients.[63] Risk factors for postoperative delirium include age, preexisting cognitive impairment or dementia, a history of delirium, and a history of alcohol dependence.[59] Several preventative strategies have been employed including use of regional anesthesia, limiting use of postoperative narcotics, rapid mobilization and return to familiar environments, and antipsychotic medications.[61,62] Medications used in preventing and treating postoperative delirium have included haloperidol, risperidone, donepezil, and olazapine.[59,61,62]

In the authors' institution appropriate at-risk patients undergoing TJR are treated prophylactically with olanzapine pre- and postoperatively, with excellent results.[62] A prospective, randomized double-blind placebo-controlled trial has demonstrated a significant reduction in postoperative delirium in these patients, with only 14% of patients in the olanzapine group experiencing postoperative delirium versus 40% of patients in the placebo group. Advanced age, higher ASA class, abnormal albumin levels, and knee replacement surgery were identified as independent risk factors for postoperative delirium.[62]

SUMMARY

Total joint arthroplasty is a safe and highly effective treatment for moderate to severe osteoarthritic symptoms and other causes of joint derangement in the elderly population. Significant improvements in pain, function, and quality of life are nearly universal, with numerous studies using validated outcome measures indicating that there is no ceiling on the age at which joint replacement surgery should be considered. Due to its success and cost-effectiveness the rate of utilization of TJR is increasing, and all health care providers must become familiar with the perioperative management of patients with joint replacements as this population continues to increase. Elderly patients may be at higher risk for postoperative medical complications; however, the majority of these are minor and the long-term results are comparable or superior to those in younger patients or age-matched population norms. As with all patients undergoing TJR, patients should be prophylactically treated for infection and thromboembolism and be carefully followed for the development of these potential complications. Postoperative delirium may be minimized and prophylactically treated in appropriate elderly patients to maximize recovery and promote safety.

REFERENCES

1. Population profile. The elderly population. Available at: http://www.census.gov/population/www/pop-profile/elderpop.html. Accessed February 26, 2010.
2. We, the American elderly. Available at: http://www.census.gov/apsd/wepeople/we-9.pdf. Accessed February 26, 2010.
3. Administration on Aging. Aging statistics. Available at: http://www.aoa.gov/aoaroot/aging_statistics/index.aspx. Accessed February 26, 2010.
4. Goldberg VM, Buckwalter JA, Hayes WC, et al. Orthopaedic challenges in an aging population. Instr Course Lect 1997;46:417–22.
5. Brummel-Smith K. Geriatrics for orthopaedics. Instr Course Lect 1997;46:409–16.
6. Day S. Geriatric orthopaedics. In: Solomon D, editor. New frontiers in the geriatrics research. New York: American Geriatric Society; 2004. p. 303.
7. Laupacis A, Bourne R, Rorabeck C, et al. The effect of elective total hip replacement on health-related quality of life. J Bone Joint Surg Am 1993;75(11):1619.
8. Ethgen O, Bruyere O, Richy F, et al. Health-related quality of life in total hip and total knee arthroplasty, a qualitative and systematic review of the literature. J Bone Joint Surg Am 2004;86(5):963–74.
9. Birdsall PD, Hayes JH, Cleary R, et al. Health outcome after total knee replacement in the very elderly. J Bone Joint Surg Br 1999;81:660–2.
10. Levy RN, Levy CM, Snyder J, et al. Outcome and long-term results following total hip replacement in elderly patients. Clin Orthop 1995;316:25–30.
11. Hamel MB, Toth M, Legedza A, et al. Joint replacement surgery in elderly patients with severe osteoarthritis of the hip or knee. Arch Intern Med 2008;168:1430–40.
12. March LM, Cross MJ, Lapsley H, et al. Outcomes after hip or knee replacement surgery for osteoarthritis: a prospective cohort study comparing patients quality of life before and after surgery with age-related population norms. Med J Aust 1999;171:235–8.
13. Hozack J, Rothman RH, Albert TJ, et al. Relationship of total hip arthroplasty outcomes to other orthopedic procedures. Clin Orthop 1997;344:81–7.
14. Lieberman JR, Dorey F, Shekelle P, et al. Outcome after total hip arthroplasty. Comparison of traditional disease-specific and a quality of life measurement of outcome. J Arthroplasty 1997;12:639–45.

15. Kiebzak GM, Vain PA, Gregory AM, et al. SF-36 general health status survey to determine patient satisfaction at short-term follow-up after total hip and knee arthroplasty. J South Orthop Assoc 1997;6:169–72.

16. Ritter MA, Albohm MJ, Keating EM, et al. Comparative outcomes of total joint arthroplasty. J Arthroplasty 1995;10:737–41.

17. Learmonth ID, Young C, Rorabeck C. The operation of the century: total hip replacement. Lancet 2007;370:1508–19.

18. Saleh KJ, Wood KC, Gafni A, et al. Immediate surgery versus waiting list policy in revision total hip arthroplasty. An economic evaluation. J Arthroplasty 1997;12:1–10.

19. Lohmander S. Osteoarthritis: a major cause of disability in the elderly. In: Buckwalter JA, Goldwater VM, Woo SLY, editors. Musculoskeletal soft-tissue aging: impact on mobility. Rosemont (IL): American Academy of Orthopaedic Surgeons; 1993. p. 99–115.

20. Hochberg MC, Altman RD, Brandt KD, et al. Guidelines for the medical management of osteoarthritis. Part I. Osteoarthritis of the hip. American College of Rheumatology. Arthritis Rheum 1995;38:1535–40.

21. Iorio R, Robb WJ, Healy WL, et al. Orthopaedic surgeon workforce and volume assessment for total hip and knee replacement in the United States: preparing for an epidemic. J Bone Joint Surg Am 2008;90:1598–605.

22. Kurtz SM, Ong KL, Schmier J, et al. Future clinical and economic impact of revision total hip and knee arthroplasty. J Bone Joint Surg Am 2007;89:144–51.

23. Kurtz SM, Ong K, Lau E, et al. Projections of primary and revision hip and knee arthroplasty in the United States from 2005 to 2030. J Bone Joint Surg Am 2007; 89:780–5.

24. Bozik KJ, Saleh KJ, Rosenberg AG, et al. Economic evaluation of total hip arthroplasty: analysis and review of the literature. J Arthroplasty 2004;19:180–9.

25. Barber T, Healy W. The hospital cost of total hip arthroplasty. J Bone Joint Surg Am 1993;75:321–5.

26. Adams ME, Atkinson MH, Lussier AJ, et al. The role of viscosupplementation with hylan G-F 20 in treatment of osteoarthritis of the knee: a Canadian multicenter trial comparing hylan G-F 20 alone, hylan G-F 20 with non-steroidal anti-inflammatory drugs and NSAIDs alone. Osteoarthritis Cartilage 1995;3:213–25.

27. Nallamshetty L, Buchowski JM, Nazarian LA, et al. Septic arthritis of the hip following cortisone injection: case report and review of the literature. Clin Imaging 2003;27(4):225–8.

28. Butler RN, Davis R, Lewis CB, et al. Physical fitness: benefits of exercise for the older patient. Geriatrics 1998;53:46–52.

29. Shah AK, Celestin J, Parks ML, et al. Long-term results of total joint arthroplasty in elderly patients who are frail. Clin Orthop 2004;425:106–9.

30. Chang RW, Pellissier JM, Hazen GB. A cost-effectiveness analysis of total hip arthroplasty for osteoarthritis of the hip. JAMA 1996;275:858–65.

31. Mahomed NN, Barrett JA, Katz JN, et al. Rates and outcomes of primary and revision total hip replacement in the United States Medicare population. J Bone Joint Surg Am 2003;85(1):27–32.

32. Petersen VS, Solgaard S, Simonsen B. Total hip replacement in patients aged 80 years and older. J Am Geriatr Soc 1989;37:219–22.

33. Brander AB, Malhotra S, Jet J, et al. Outcome of hip and knee arthroplasty in persons aged 80 years and older. Clin Orthop 1997;345:67–78.

34. Jones CA, Voaklander DC, Johnston WC, et al. The effect of age on pain, function, and quality of life after total hip and knee arthroplasty. Arch Intern Med 2001;161:454–60.

35. Zicat B, Rorabeck CH, Bourne RB, et al. Total knee arthroplasty in the octogenarian. J Arthroplasty 1993;8:395–400.
36. Pettine KA, Aamlid BC, Cabanela ME. Elective total hip arthroplasty in patients older than 80 years of age. Clin Orthop 1991;266:127–32.
37. Keisu KS, Orozco F, Sharkey PF, et al. Primary cementless total hip arthroplasty in octogenarians. Two to eleven-year follow-up. J Bone Joint Surg Am 2001;83(3): 359–63.
38. Katz BP, Freund DA, Heck DA, et al. Demographic variation in the rate of knee replacement: a multi-year analysis. Health Serv Res 1996;31:125–40.
39. Hernandez-Vaquero D, Fernandez-Carreira JM, Perez-Hernandez D, et al. Total knee arthroplasty in the elderly. Is there an age limit? J Arthroplasty 2006;21: 358–61.
40. Biau D, Mullins MM, Judet T, et al. Is anyone too old for a total knee replacement? Clin Orthop 2006;448:180–4.
41. Karuppiah SV, Banaszkiewicz PA, Ledingham WM. The mortality, morbidity and cost benefits of elective total knee arthroplasty in the nonagenarian population. Int Orthop 2008;32:339–43.
42. Adam RF, Noble J. Primary total knee arthroplasty in the elderly. J Arthroplasty 1994;9:495–7.
43. Hosick WB, Lotke PA, Baldwin A. Total knee arthroplasty in patients 80 years of age and older. Clin Orthop 1994;299:77–80.
44. Newington DP, Bannister GC, Fordyce M. Primary total hip replacement in patients over 80 years of age. J Bone Joint Surg Br 1990;72:450–2.
45. Phillips TW, Grainger RW, Cameron HS, et al. Risks and benefits of elective hip replacement in the octogenarian. CMAJ 1987;137:497–500.
46. Berry DJ, von Knoch M, Schleck CD, et al. The cumulative long-term risk of dislocation after primary Charnley total hip arthroplasty. J Bone Joint Surg Am 2004; 86(1):9–14.
47. Mantilla CB, Horlocker TT, Schroeder DR, et al. Frequency of myocardial infarction, pulmonary embolism, deep venous thrombosis and death following primary hip or knee arthroplasty. Anesthesiology 2002;96(5):1140–6.
48. Lee J, Singletary R, Schmader K, et al. Surgical site infection in the elderly following orthopaedic surgery, risk factors and outcomes. J Bone Joint Surg Am 2006;88:1705–12.
49. Kurtz SM, Ong KL, Lau E, et al. Prosthetic joint infection risk after TKA in the Medicare population. Clin Orthop 2010;468:52–6.
50. Leone JM, Hanssen AD. Management of infection at the site of a total knee arthroplasty. J Bone Joint Surg Am 2005;87:2335–48.
51. Peersman G, Laskin R, Davis G, et al. Infection in knee replacement: a retrospective review of 6489 total knee replacements. Clin Orthop 2001;392: 15–23.
52. Pulido L, Ghanem E, Joshi A, et al. Periprosthetic joint infection: the incidence, timing and predisposing factors. Clin Orthop 2008;466(7):1710–5.
53. Patel VP, Walsh M, Sehgal B, et al. Factors associated with prolonged wound drainage after primary total hip and knee arthroplasty. J Bone Joint Surg Am 2007;89(1):33–8.
54. Jamsen E, Huhtala H, Puolakka T, et al. Risk factors for infection after knee arthroplasty, a register-based analysis of 43,149 cases. J Bone Joint Surg Am 2009; 91(1):38–47.
55. Masterson EL, Masri BA, Duncan CP. Treatment of infection at the site of total hip replacement. J Bone Joint Surg Am 1997;79:1740–9.

56. Lieberman JR, Hsu WK. Prevention of venous thromboembolic disease after total hip and knee arthroplasty. J Bone Joint Surg Am 2005;87:2097–112.

57. Johanson NA, Lachiewicz PF, Lieberman JR, et al. Prevention of symptomatic pulmonary embolism in patients undergoing total hip or knee arthroplasty. J Am Acad Orthop Surg 2009;17(3):183–96.

58. Bern M, Deshmukh RV, Nelso R, et al. Low-dose warfarin coupled with lower leg compression is effective prophylaxis against thromboembolic disease after hip arthroplasty. J Arthroplasty 2007;22:644–50.

59. Inouye SK. Delirium in older persons. N Engl J Med 2006;354:1157–65.

60. Robinson TN, Raeburn CD, Tran ZV, et al. Postoperative delirium in the elderly: risk factors and outcomes. Ann Surg 2009;249:173–8.

61. Sampson EL, Raven PR, Ndhlovu PN, et al. A randomized, double-blind, placebo-controlled trial of donepezil hydrochloride (Aricept) for reducing the incidence of postoperative delirium after elective total hip replacement. Int J Geriatr Psychiatry 2007;22:343–9.

62. Larsen KA, Kelly SE, Stern TA, et al. Administration of olanzapine to prevent postoperative delirium in the elderly joint replacement patient: a randomized controlled trial. Psychosomatics 2010, in press.

63. Leslie DL, Marcantonio ER, Zhang Y, et al. One-year health care costs associated with delirium in the elderly population. Arch Intern Med 2008;168:27–32.

INDEX

Note: Page numbers of article titles are in **boldface** type.

Clin Geriatr Med 26 (2010) 531–538
doi:10.1016/S0749-0690(10)00063-7
0749-0690/10/$ – see front matter © 2010 Elsevier Inc. All rights reserved.

geriatric.theclinics.com

O

Moving?

Make sure your subscription moves with you!

To notify us of your new address, find your **Clinics Account Number** (located on your mailing label above your name), and contact customer service at:

Email: journalscustomerservice-usa@elsevier.com

800-654-2452 (subscribers in the U.S. & Canada)
314-447-8871 (subscribers outside of the U.S. & Canada)

Fax number: 314-447-8029

Elsevier Health Sciences Division
Subscription Customer Service
3251 Riverport Lane
Maryland Heights, MO 63043

*To ensure uninterrupted delivery of your subscription, please notify us at least 4 weeks in advance of move.

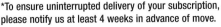